Chronic Lung Diseases

Sheikh Rayees • Inshah Din •
Gurdarshan Singh • Fayaz A. Malik
Editors

Chronic Lung Diseases

Pathophysiology and Therapeutics

Springer

Editors
Sheikh Rayees
Department of Pharmacology
University of Illinois at Chicago
Illinois, IL, USA

Inshah Din
Department of Biochemistry
University of Kashmir
Srinagar, Jammu and Kashmir, India

Gurdarshan Singh
Toxicology
CSIR-IIM
Jammu, Jammu and Kashmir, India

Fayaz A. Malik
Cancer Pharmacology
CSIR-IIM
Jammu, Jammu and Kashmir, India

ISBN 978-981-15-3733-2 ISBN 978-981-15-3734-9 (eBook)
https://doi.org/10.1007/978-981-15-3734-9

This Springer imprint is published by the registered company Springer Nature Singapore Pte Ltd.
The registered company address is: 152 Beach Road, #21-01/04 Gateway East, Singapore 189721, Singapore

Contents

About the Editors

Sheikh Rayees is a pharmacologist working at the University of Illinois at Chicago, USA. He completed his M.Sc. in Biotechnology at HNB Garhwal University (a Central University) followed by his doctoral degree at the prestigious CSIR-Indian Institute of Integrative Medicine and SMVDU, Jammu, India. Mr. Rayees is currently working towards understanding the biology and therapeutics of respiratory disorders like acute lung injury and acute respiratory distress syndrome. He has published several articles in leading peer-reviewed journals and has sound academic credentials. Mr. Rayees received several awards throughout his doctoral and postdoctoral research career.

Inshah Din is a research scholar working at Govt. Medical College, Srinagar. She completed her M.Sc. in Clinical Biochemistry, followed by an M.Phil. and Ph.D. in Biochemistry at the University of Kashmir. She has worked as a Junior Research fellow at the prestigious Sher-i-Kashmir Institute of Medical Sciences, Srinagar. Ms. Din has sound academic credentials and has published several research articles in peer-reviewed journals.

Gurdarshan Singh is a pharmacologist working as a principal scientist at the prestigious CSIR-Indian Institute of Integrative Medicine. He completed his M. Sc., M.Phil., and Ph.D. at Jammu University, India. Mr. Gurdarshan is currently Head of the PK-PD Toxicology Division at the CSIR-Indian Institute of Integrative Medicine, Jammu. His main research interests include evaluating new and potent drug-like molecules for their safety pharmacology, pharmacodynamic and pharmacokinetic properties. He has worked in several areas of preclinical research, e.g., asthma, hypertension, and cancer. Dr. Singh holds several patents and contributed to the development of Risorine, an antituberculosis drug and the world's first boosted-rifampicin treatment with a fixed-dose combination.

Fayaz A. Malik is an Indian cancer biologist and pharmacologist at the prestigious CSIR-Indian Institute of Integrative Medicine. He is known for his studies on investigating the regulatory mechanisms of cancer stem cells during tumor metastasis. He has also studied the identification of signaling networks that confer resistance to current anticancer therapies. The Department of Biotechnology of the Government of India awarded him the National Bioscience Award for Career Development, one of the most coveted Indian science awards, for his contributions to biosciences in 2014. In addition, the Department of Science and Technology of the Government of India awarded him the Swarnajayanti Fellowship, one of the most prestigious fellowship awards, for his advanced research in cancer biology.

Therapeutic Advances in the Management of Pulmonary Arterial Hypertension

1

Suyeon Heo, Nancy Ly, Madeeha Aqil, Mohd Shahid, M. Rizwan Siddiqui, Zulfiqar Ahmad, and Mohammad Tauseef

Abstract

Pulmonary arterial hypertension (PAH) is a progressive disease with multiple etiologies. If remains untreated, it leads to high rate of morbidity and mortality, and a median survival of only 5–7 years. Clinically, PAH is defined as mean pulmonary arterial pressure >20 mmHg at rest with normal left atrial pressure. PAH is characterized by remodeling of the pulmonary vasculature due to pulmonary vascular endothelial and smooth cell proliferation. These events eventually reduce the pulmonary arterial compliance and thus causing increased pulmonary vascular resistance. If remains unmanaged, it will ultimately end up in right ventricular failure. However, the Food and Drug Administration (FDA) has approved drugs that target the endothelial pathway, the nitric oxide pathway, and the prostacyclin pathway. These therapeutic strategies, mainly inducing pulmonary vasodilation, however, have poor effect on the signaling pathways activated during the pathogenesis of PAH. This might be one of the reasons why they are unable to reverse the pathology of the disease, and eventually patients stop responding to them. If medications fail, the only viable alternative will be lung transplantation to save a patient's life. Evidences show the contribution of

S. Heo · N. Ly · M. Shahid · M. Tauseef (✉)
Department of Pharmaceutical Sciences, Chicago State University College of Pharmacy, Chicago, IL, USA
e-mail: mtauseef@csu.edu

M. Aqil
Freelance Medical Writer, American Medical Writers Association (AMWA), Rockville, MD, USA

M. R. Siddiqui
Department of Pediatrics, Northwestern University Feinberg School of Medicine, Chicago, IL, USA

Z. Ahmad
Department of Biochemistry, Kirksville College of Osteopathic Medicine, A.T. Still University, Kirksville, MO, USA

S. Rayees et al. (eds.), *Chronic Lung Diseases*,
https://doi.org/10.1007/978-981-15-3734-9_1

heredity, inflammation, drugs, toxins, HIV infection, and hepatic diseases in the progression of PAH. Therefore, there is a need for potential therapeutics, which, via affecting the pathological signaling pathways, halt the disease process and eventually reverse the pulmonary remodeling in the patients. In this chapter, we discuss the emerging novel therapeutics and their mechanism of actions, which have advanced beyond preclinical research and are currently being investigated in the clinical cases of PAH.

Keywords

Pulmonary arterial hypertension · Vascular smooth muscle proliferation · Clinical trials · Lung inflammation · Bone morphogenetic protein receptor 2 (BMPR2) · Hypoxia · Endothelial cells · Pulmonary artery

1.1 Introduction

The pulmonary hypertension is defined as elevated pulmonary arterial pressure (PAP) [1–4]. It is characterized by pulmonary vascular remodeling in the small pulmonary arteries, increased PAP and elevated pulmonary vascular resistance (PVR) [5]. The etiology of pulmonary hypertension (PH) is multifactorial [1, 6]. Other noticeable changes during the development of PH include intimal proliferation, vascular smooth muscle proliferation or hypertrophy, and adventitial thickening [7, 8]. The symptoms of the disease are progressive such as shortness of breath, fatigue, chest discomfort, abdominal fullness, and light-headedness or even syncope with more advanced and severe form of the disease [9, 10]. If remain untreated, or uncontrolled by the currently available medications, patients of PH will eventually need heart and lung transplantation. Otherwise, it leads to increased rate of mortality [5, 11]. Thus, PH is emerging as an urgent medical need, which requires a thorough understating of its pathogenesis at cellular and molecular levels, and thereby development of potential novel therapeutics to treat the PH [1, 2, 6].

Several confounding factors, including aberrations in the genes, environmental toxins, drugs, hepatic disease, and right heart dysfunction, to mention but a few, are involved in the pathogenesis of PH [3, 12]. Clinically, PH is a mean pulmonary arterial pressure more than 25 mmHg determined by resting supine right heart catheterization (RHC) [9, 11, 13]. According to the current classification and criteria [13], PH may be categorized into (1) idiopathic, which is defined by the absence of underlying risk factor, (2) heritable/genetic, for instance, the presence of germline mutation in bone morphogenetic protein receptor 2 (*BMPR2*), (3) PH induced by drugs or toxins, or (4) it may be associated with other pathological conditions such as connective tissue disease, portal hypertension, HIV infections, and congenital heart disease. The most updated PH classification was defined at the 5th World Symposium on Pulmonary Hypertension in 2013 [3, 13]. This classification is based on a shared disease histology and pathophysiology, clinical presentation and therapeutic interventions. Thus, this put the PH in five differed groups: (1) pulmonary arterial hypertension (PAH), (2) PH due to left heart disease or pulmonary venous hypertension, (3) PH due to chronic lung disease and/or hypoxia, (4) chronic thromboembolic PH (CTEPH), and (5) PH due to undefined or unknown mechanism [9, 12].

1.2 Basic Review of Pulmonary Circulation

The basic understanding of physiology and pathophysiology of pulmonary circulation will be helpful to better understand and define the pathogenesis, diagnosis, prognosis, and therapeutic aspects of the PH. Briefly, the major function of the pulmonary circulation is to carry deoxygenated blood from the right side of the heart to the lungs via pulmonary artery to get it oxygenated [13, 14] and return oxygen-rich blood back to the left side of the heart via pulmonary vain. Therefore, maintenance of pulmonary circulation function is vital to provide oxygenated blood to the systemic circulation [12].

The pulmonary arterial hypertension (PAH) is a progressive process that leads to an increase in pulmonary vascular resistance, and is a most common type of PH in clinical practice. This is due to the multiple pathophysiologic outcomes such as pulmonary vascular remodeling and sustained vasoconstriction. Since pulmonary circulation is getting the entire cardiac output, low pressure and PVR in the pulmonary artery are maintained through the high cross-sectional area containing network of small pulmonary arteries and capillaries. One may predict that any change or fluctuation in the PVR will be reflected in the increase in pulmonary arterial pressure and leads to PH. Anatomically, the pulmonary artery is comprised of three distinct types of tissue layers. The innermost intima is comprised of pulmonary artery endothelial cells, followed by the middle layer of media containing pulmonary artery smooth muscle cells. The outermost layer or lining is made of the fibrous tissue called adventitia. In the pathogenesis of PH, the above cell types play a fundamental role in causing narrowing of the pulmonary artery and increasing PVR. The current line of therapeutics mostly targets proliferation of intimal and medial cells proliferation but is unable to reverse the disease progression (Fig. 1.1) [6, 12, 14].

1.3 Pulmonary Hypertension: Clinical Classification

Under clinical setting, PH is more of comorbid condition, which is most of the time associated with other types of clinical conditions. This makes a poor prognosis and ends up in high rate of morbidity and mortality [2, 12, 14]. This puts a great challenge on clinicians and pulmonary physician to correctly diagnose the disease. Over the past several years, a great stride has been done to improve the understanding of the pathophysiology of the PH. One of the challenging tasks is to correctly classify the disease based on the pathophysiological origin of the disease. Here, we will expand the classification of PH so that we may be able to better understand the disease process. In 1970, the efforts led by the World Health Organization (WHO)

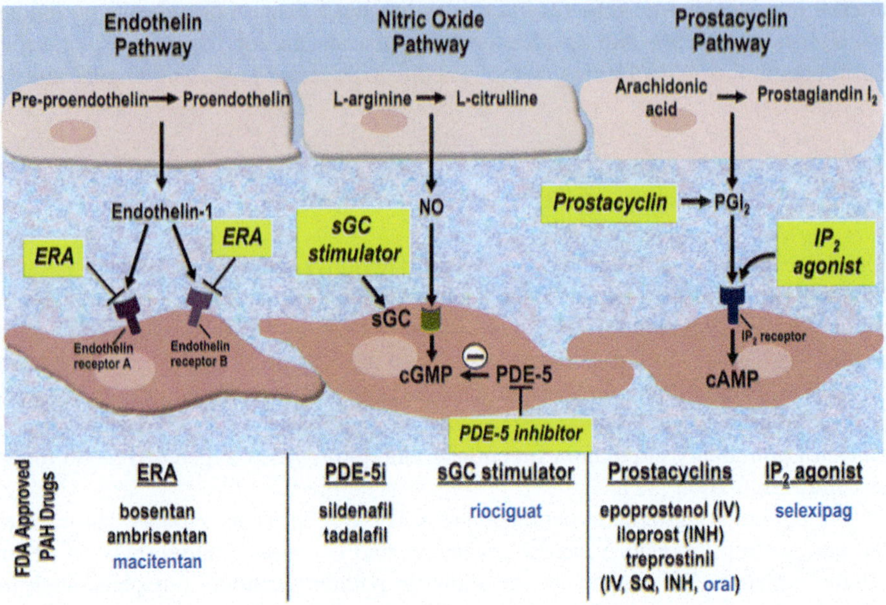

Fig. 1.1 Pathways targeted in current therapies for pulmonary arterial hypertension. Newly approved therapies are listed in blue. *cAMP* cyclic adenosine monophosphate, *cGMP* cyclic guanylate monophosphate, *ERA* endothelin receptor antagonist, *FDA* US Food and Drug Administration, *INH* inhaled, *IP2* prostacyclin receptor 2, *IV* intravenous, *NO* nitric oxide, *PAH* pulmonary arterial hypertension, *PDE-5* phosphodiesterase-5, *PDE-5i* phosphodiesterase-5 inhibitor, *PGI2* prostaglandin I2, *sGC* soluble guanylate cyclase, *SQ* subcutaneous. (Reproduced with permission from Tsai H, Sung YK and de Jesus Perez V. Recent advances in the management of pulmonary arterial hypertension [version 1]. F1000Research 2016, 5:2755 [6])

resulted in the understanding of the underlying causes of PH. This further led to putting PH as primary or secondary PH. This was the beginning of the understanding of the tip of the iceberg basically, which opened doors for the further discoveries in the field of PH. The most current and updated PH classifications were defined at the 5th World Symposium on PH in 2013 and put the pH cases in five separate types, as defined above [12, 14]. Now the question is: What was the outcome on the patients' overall health and survival in PH? The above classification system impacted significantly on the patients' diagnosis and treatment process due to more focused identification of the factors affecting morbidity and mortality in PH [12, 13].

The question which is still vaguely answered is why the diagnosis of PH is so challenging. There is no single and clear answer to this question. One of the most important challenges with the diagnosis of PH is that the early symptoms of the disease are nonspecific and that may lead to misdiagnosis [6, 15]. This may require more intensive physical examination and may be more invasive clinical procedures to delineate the disease in patients at early stage [8, 16].

Patients with PH displayed varying symptoms starting from unexplained dyspnea upon exertion, chest pain, fatigue, hemoptysis, syncope, and Raynaud's phenomena.

These symptoms most of the time are poor oxygen transport and impaired cardiac output due to the increased pulmonary vascular resistance. Therefore, only a thorough clinical investigation may reveal the underlying pathophysiology pertinent to PH. Other signs, which were revealed upon clinical examination, include jugular venous distensions, hepatomegaly, cyanosis, the presence of hepatojugular reflex, mottled extremities, diminished peripheral pulses, peripheral edema, and ascites [12, 16]. Cardiac catheterization is a reliable mode to delineate and differentiate multiple abnormal sounds associated with pulmonary artery hypertension such as RV, S3 and S4 sounds, accentuated pulmonic valve component (P2) of the second heart sound, systolic murmur suggesting pulmonary regurgitation, and a parasternal lift may be detectable [12]. This indicates how rigorously patient should be examined to reach at a conclusion, from where the medications will be initiated [12, 16].

Besides what is explained above, other invasive and noninvasive techniques are further required at the final stage for the explicit diagnostic purpose of PH. These include electrocardiography, pulmonary function testing, chest radiography, echocardiography, serologic testing, and right heart catheterization [12]. With such an advancement of the diagnostic technology in PH, it is a fact that the current therapeutics, which is being used at the clinic, is merely a supportive care that targets pulmonary vasocontraction. At this point, we may ask a question why at the verge of advancement of medical technology, we are feeling so helpless therapeutically and relying on conjecture rather than really treating or reversing the disease. The answer is maybe either we are still lacking the correct understanding of pathological process that takes place at the cellular and molecular level or we need to develop rationale drugs that target the disease at the cellular and molecular level. We will discuss the advancement in these areas in forthcoming paragraphs. First, we will briefly review the different types of PH [1, 16].

1.3.1 Group 1: Pulmonary Arterial Hypertension (PAH)

Group 1 pulmonary hypertension or pulmonary arterial hypertension (PAH) is a progressively increased pressure in the pulmonary artery or increase in mean pulmonary arterial pressure (Fig. 1.2) [6, 8, 12]. Primarily, it is due to the proliferation of vascular smooth muscle in the pulmonary artery, which leads to the obstruction in the blood flow in pulmonary vasculature. If it remains untreated, it will eventually end up in right ventricular failure and often cause premature death. In terms of the etiology, there are multiple factors involved in the progression of the disease and few of them are well understood. For instance, in idiopathic pulmonary hypertension, we do not have any clear understanding of the etiology of the disease. Other important factors which are involved include heredity, drug-induced PAH, various connective tissue-related abnormalities, human immunodeficiency virus, or HIV infection, and congenital abnormities in the heart. PAH may also arise following other vasculo-occlusive disorders including portal hypertension, veno-occlusive diseases and persistent pulmonary hypertension of the newborns. It was a time when there was a lack of therapeutics and the median life span oftentimes was less than

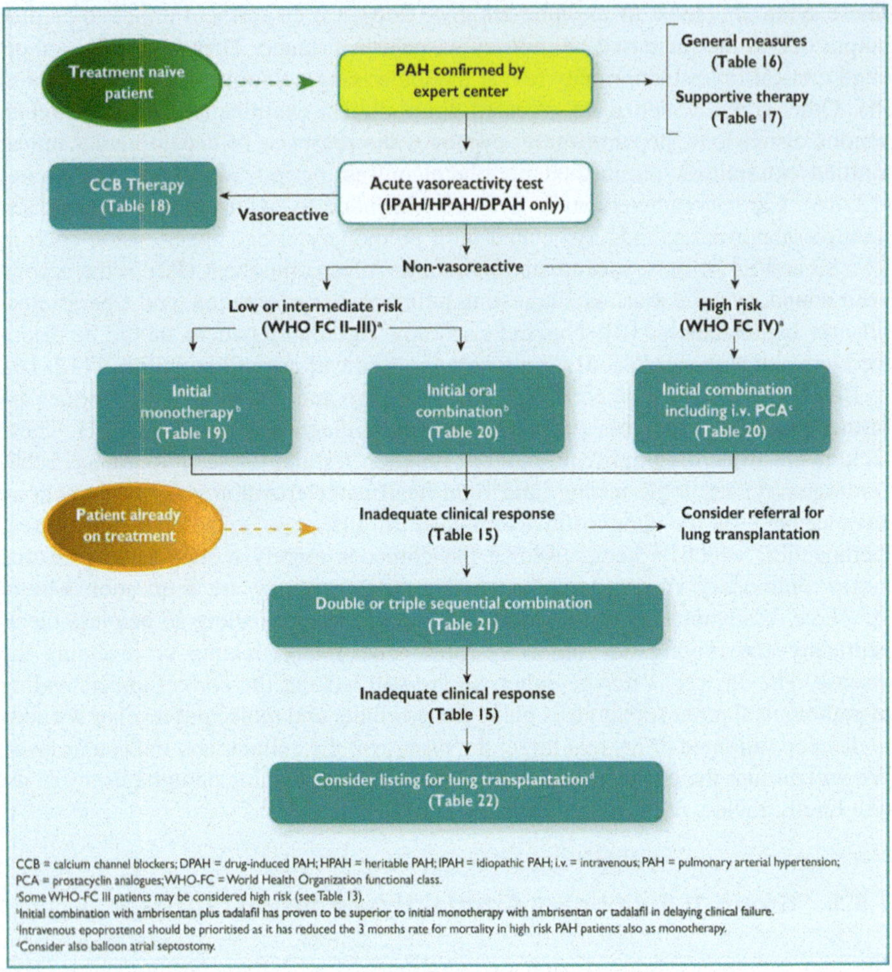

Fig. 1.2 Treatment algorithm from the 2015 European Society of Cardiology/European Respiratory Society guidelines for the diagnosis and treatment of pulmonary hypertension. (Reproduced with permission from Tsai H, Sung YK and de Jesus Perez V. Recent advances in the management of pulmonary arterial hypertension [version 1]. F1000Research 2016, 5:2755 [6])

3 years [12, 17]. With the advent of more targeted therapies, along with the early diagnosis of the disease, the clinical outcome is much improved. Recent research demonstrates involvement of gene mutation and development of PAH. For instance, mutation in the bone morphogenetic protein receptor 2 (BMPR2) gene has been involved in more than 75% cases of clinically diagnosed PAH. Intriguingly, these cases mostly have a known family history of PAH. There are up to 25% of sporadic cases with more than 300 known independent mutations in the gene alone [12, 18]. This suggests that mutated BMPR2 is the most commonly involved denominator in the pathogenesis of PAH. The mutated gene product binds and

activates members of the transforming growth factor (TGF)-β family, including activin-like receptor kinase-1 (ALK-1), endoglin (ENG), and mothers against decapentaplegic homolog 9 (SMAd9) have also been identified in the etiology of the PAH. This suggests a significant role of this signaling cascade in the development of PAH [19]. Besides the clear central role of TGF-β family, recent studies indicate mutations in caveolin-1 (CAV-1) and potassium two pore domain channel subfamily K member 3 (KCNK3) has a significant role in the etiology and pathogenesis of PAH [19, 20].

Research studies demonstrate the potential role of drugs and toxins in the pathology of PAH [19, 21, 22]. However, exactly how these chemical compounds lead to PAH is still in obscurity. Very few drugs and chemicals have been known so far, which cause PAH with some defined understanding. Under these categories, for instance, certain anorexigens (e.g., aminorex, fenfluramine, and dexfenfluramine), toxic rapeseed oil, selective serotonin inhibitors (SSRIs) and benfluorex cause PAH in the patients. Although the precise mechanism of anorexigens in inducing PAH is unclear, studies show that they basically block the uptake of serotonin via blocking the serotonin transporter [1, 12, 15]. This allows serotonin to induce proliferation of pulmonary vascular smooth cells and induction of PAH. Benflurex shares an active metabolite with fenfluramine, and is a drug used in Europe to treat hyperglycemia and other metabolic disorders, causing PAH. Moreover, SSRIs are used in pregnancy, and increase the risk of PAH. It also increases the risk of mortality and worsening the PAH if used in patients who are already diagnosed with PAH [12, 21, 22].

Other drugs that have strong link to induce PAH include amphetamine, methamphetamine, L-tryptophan, dasatinib, cocaine, phenylpropanolamine, St. John's wort, chemotherapeutic agents, and interferon α and β [23]. However, there is no strong relation between cigarette smoking, estrogens, or oral contraceptives in the induction of PAH [12, 23].

1.3.2 Group 2: Pulmonary Hypertension (PH) Due to Left Heart Disease

Group 2 PH due to left heart disease includes left ventricular (LV) diastolic dysfunction, left ventricular (LV) systolic dysfunction, valvular disease, congenital and or acquired left heart inflow/outflow tract obstruction, and congenital cardiomyopathies (25 and current) [24]. Most common presence of group 2 PH has been observed in the patients suffering heart failure with reduced (HFeEF) or preserved ejection fraction (HFpEF). Hemodynamically, the disease is defined as mean pulmonary arterial pressure (mPAP) $\geq$ 25 mmHg, a pulmonary artery wedge pressure (PAWP) or left ventricular end-diastolic pressure (LVEDP) $>$ 15 mmHg, and a normal or reduced cardiac output [12]. The pathophysiological manifestation involved the passive backward transmission of filling pressures that increases mPAP (e.g., loss of left atrial compliance, diastolic dysfunction, mitral valve regurgitation), further increase in mPAP (e.g., endothelial dysfunction, vasoconstriction), and eventually ends up in worsening of pulmonary vascular remodeling, right ventricular dysfunction and, if remain untreatable, ultimately leads to high rate of mortality [12, 24].

Group 2 PH is further categorized into two sub categories. This subclassification is based on the diastolic pressure difference (DPD, defined as [diastolic PAP – mean PAWP]) during right heart catheterization under resting conditions. These categories are isolated post capillary PH (PAWP $>$ 15 mmHg and DPD $<$ 15 mmHg) and combined post and precapillary PH (PAWP $>$ 15 mmHg and DPD $\geq$ 7 mmHg) [12, 24].

The clinical features of Group 2 PH are different compared to Group 1 PAH. Group 2 PH patients with HFpEF were older in age, superimposed with other cardiovascular comorbidities such as hypertension, coronary artery disease, worse exercise capacity, and renal dysfunction [25]. They were also suffering from high frequency of left atrial enlargement, lower frequency of right atrial enlargement and less severe PH. Therapeutically, there is more focus to treat the underlying heart disease present in Group 2 PH to achieve desirable effects [12, 24].

1.3.3 Group 3: Pulmonary Hypertension (PH) Due to Lung Diseases and Hypoxia

The pathological conditions associated with the underlying cause of Group 3 PH include chronic obstructive pulmonary disease (COPD), interstitial lung disease (ILD) (e.g., idiopathic pulmonary fibrosis, sarcoidosis), and other lung diseases such as with the involvement of sleep disorder-induced breathing problems, alveolar hyperventilation disorders, chronic high-altitude exposure, and developmental lung diseases [12, 26]. Since there is an increased propensity of above associated pulmonary disorders, sometimes, it is very difficult to distinguish the differences between idiopathic PAH and Group 3 PH. At the diagnostic end, findings suggest that the Group 3 PH is associated with moderate-to-severe impairment in ventilation function, reduced breathing reserve, and characteristic airway and/or parenchymal abnormalities [12].

Two significant pathophysiological features underlying Group 3 PH include hypoxic vasoconstriction and obliteration of the pulmonary vascular bed. Hypoxia leads to a significant damage to the vasculature and release of vasoconstrictor substance such as endothelin from the endothelium. Upon release, endothelin causes underlying vascular smooth muscle cell contraction and leads to vasoconstriction and proliferation. Initial hypoxia-induced vasoconstriction is reversible; however, once there is pulmonary remodeling due to the chronic hypoxic condition, it is largely irreversible. Like Group 2 PH, Group 3 PH management also involves identification and treatment of underlying pathophysiologic cause rather than only focusing on the increased in mPAP [12].

1.3.4 Group 4: Chronic Thromboembolic PH (CTEPH)

Group 4 pulmonary hypertension is due to the chronic thromboembolic disease that leads to prolonged occlusion of the pulmonary vasculature [27]. This disease arises due to the abnormal activation of blood coagulation cascade in the vasculature. Pathologically, there is an abnormality at the level of fibrinolysis or any underlying hematological or autoimmune disorders ultimately leading to the hypercoagulable state and poor resolution of thrombosis. Group 4 PH is manageable through surgical intervention along with drug therapy. In this unique situation, through pulmonary thromboendarterectomy, a surgeon removes chronic blood clots from the pulmonary artery. Long-term anticoagulation medicines are recommended [27, 28].

1.3.5 Group 5: PH with Unclear Multifactorial Mechanism

Group 5 PH includes all the clinical conditions of PH where there are unclear multifactorial mechanisms of the disease origin. This category includes hematologic disorders (sickle cell disease), β-thalassemia, chronic hemolytic anemia, myeloproliferative disorders, splenectomy, metabolic disorders (glycogen storage disease, Gaucher disease, and thyroid disorders), and systemic disorders (sarcoidosis, lymphangioleiomyomatosis, and pulmonary histiocytosis). Post capillary PH in sickle cell disease is secondary to left ventricular dysfunction, whereas precapillary PH may cause by vasculopathy from the intravascular hemolysis, chronic pulmonary thromboembolism, or enhanced activity of pulmonary hypoxic response [29]. This category is so far the most poorly studied type of PH. The reason is its multimechanism activation etiology. Therefore, to well characterize this class, further research is warranted. So far, there is a serious lack of underrating of its pathology [29].

1.4 Mechanisms of Pathogenesis and Pathophysiology of Pulmonary Hypertension

As we consistently noted in the previous sections of this chapter, the main vascular changes in all forms of the pulmonary hypertension are vasoconstriction, smooth muscle cell proliferation, and even thrombosis. These pathological findings suggest an imbalance between vasodilation and vasoconstriction mechanisms [6, 15]. They also indicate perturbations even at the level of growth inhibitors and mitogenic factors and cause more inclination toward the prothrombotic state and alteration in the antithrombotic milieu. Hence, these off-balance homeostatic processes may ultimately lead to pulmonary endothelial dysfunction and injury [6, 15, 30].

1.4.1 Prostacyclin and Thromboxane A_2

Prostacyclin and thromboxane A_2 are potent vasodilator and vasoconstrictor, respectively [31]. They are generated in the vascular tissue during arachidonic acid metabolism. In contrast to the thromboxane A_2, prostacyclin inhibits platelets aggregation and prevents smooth muscle proliferation [31]. In the pulmonary hypertension, there is abundance in the generation of thromboxane A_2 compared to prostacyclin, and henceforth, pulmonary vasoconstriction, smooth muscle proliferation, and initiation of the process of thrombosis [32]. Moreover, it was observed that the generation of prostacyclin has been reduced in the small and medium-sized pulmonary arteries of the patients diagnosed with pulmonary hypertension, especially cases of the idiopathic pulmonary arterial hypertension [30].

1.4.2 Endothelin-1

Endothelin-1 is produced by the endothelial cells and is a powerful vasoconstrictor. It stimulates the pulmonary artery smooth muscle proliferation. Plasma levels of the endothelin-1 have been found to be increased in the patients of pulmonary hypertension [33]. The levels of the endothelin-1 are found to be inversely proportional to the degree of the pulmonary vascular blood flow and the cardiac output [34]. These important observations suggest a significant role of the endothelin-1 in the pathophysiologic hemodynamic changes that occur in patients of pulmonary hypertension [9, 30].

1.4.3 Nitric Oxide

Nitric Oxide (NO) is similar to Endothelin-1 produced by the endothelial cells; however, it induces a vasodilation via relaxing the vascular smooth muscle of the pulmonary vasculature [35]. It also inhibits pulmonary smooth muscle proliferation and prevents the platelets aggregation. The synthesis of the NO in the endothelial cell is regulated by the family of the enzymes, nitric oxide synthase (NOS). Studies show the decreased levels of the NOS in the pulmonary vessel of patients of pulmonary hypertension [36]. Thus, this sets the stage for pulmonary endothelial dysfunction, smooth muscle proliferation, and prothrombotic state [30, 36].

1.4.4 Serotonin

Serotonin, a 5-hydroxythryptamine, is vasoconstrictor and induces a smooth muscle cell proliferation [37, 38]. Due to the defect in the platelets that leads to hampered uptake of serotonin in platelets, it has been found to be involved in the pathogenesis of pulmonary hypertension. Research studies have described the genetic mutation in the serotonin transporter (5-HTT) and 5-hydroxytryptamine 2B receptor (5HT2B) in the platelets, which is associated with pulmonary arterial hypertension [37, 38]. However, other studies have observed that selective serotonin-reuptake inhibitors (SSRIs) increase the serotonin via inhibiting the serotonin transport, are rather protective in the setting of hypoxia, and not increasing the pulmonary hypertension. Thus, it may suggest that the levels of the serotonin itself may not be the only determinant of pulmonary hypertension. Therefore, more research is required to delineate the exact role of serotonin in the pathogenies of pulmonary hypertension [30].

1.4.5 Vasoactive Intestinal Peptide

Vasoactive intestinal peptide (VIP) is a powerful vasodilator and decreases pulmonary artery pressure and vascular resistance [10, 39]. It also has inhibitory effects on the platelet aggregation and suppresses smooth muscle proliferation. Clinical study showed the decreased levels of VIP in the serum and in the lungs of the patients of pulmonary arterial hypertension [10, 39]. However, providing inhalation therapy of VIP to the patients improved the symptoms and the hemodynamic alterations in the patients of pulmonary hypertension [6, 30].

1.4.6 Vascular Endothelial Growth Factors

Both acute hypoxia and chronic hypoxia lead to increased secretions of vascular endothelial growth factors (VEGF) along with increased expression of VEGF receptors, VEGF receptor-1 (KDR/flk) and VEGF receptor-2 (flt) in the lungs. Increased VEGF signaling in pulmonary arterial hypertension may be involved in abrupt angiogenesis, an underlying cause of the formation of the plexiform lesions and the clonal expression of the endothelial cells within the lesions [30, 40].

The above observations show that there is a clear inclination toward an increased vascular constriction response, enhanced vascular smooth muscle cell proliferation, and thrombosis [41]. Current treatment strategies are focused on bringing back the vascular and coagulation imbalances toward normalcy [34]. For instance, the therapeutic strategies developed based upon above observations, such as vasodilator prostaglandin analogue, epiprotenol, endothelial-derived relaxing factor, nitric oxide (NO), and endothelial-derived vasoconstrictor, and endothelin receptor antagonists, have been in the clinic to improve hemodynamic responses in pulmonary vascular [42]. Presently, there are important therapeutic approaches available to manage pulmonary arterial and idiopathic pulmonary hypertension in patients. They significantly increase the life expectancy of patients [42]. However, on the flip side, these medications have their own cons such as they have strong side effects profile, and most of the time patients stop to respond to these medications. And eventually, they need heart or lung transplantation [41]. Therefore, without any ambiguity, pulmonary hypertension is an unmet medical need, which warrants the development of newer therapeutics to target the disease. Recent studies suggest the emergence of the newer and improved therapeutic approaches to manage the pulmonary arterial hypertension [30, 40]. In the next sections, we will discuss the newer medications and their mechanisms of action in detail.

1.5 Emerging Therapeutics in the Management of Pulmonary Arterial Hypertension

The prevalence of all forms of the pulmonary hypertension (PH) is approximately about 15–50 per million individuals, with a prevalence of 2.4 per million per year [2, 9]. Studies further show that for the different forms of pulmonary arterial hypertension (PAH), such as idiopathic PH or heritable PH, female sex ratio is emerging as a risk factor. Out of the total cases of PAH, 80% are women. PH causes approximately about 15% risk of mortality within 1 year and 30% risk of death within 3 years in poorly controlled patients. One of the reasons for the poor prognosis of the disease may be incomplete understanding of the underlying pathophysiology of the disease. Newer and emerging therapies targeting the novel disease pathways discovered in the pathogenies of the disease will be discussed hereunder [1, 9].

For the last two decades, there is significant improvement in the treatment strategies of PH. US Food and Drug Administration (FDA) has approved 14 newer therapies to be delivered via oral, inhaled, subcutaneous, and intravenous routes to target the three potential established pathological pathways involved in the progression of pulmonary arterial hypertension. These pathways are endothelin, prostacyclin, and nitric oxide-mediated pulmonary vascular homeostasis (Fig. 1.1) [6]. Besides, investigators have pursued and identified new mechanistic pathways with novel interventions to halt the disease progression in difficult-to-manage conditions (Fig. 1.1) [1, 4, 6, 43].

1.5.1 Sex Hormones

Since women are more affected with PH than man, multicentered, international, preclinical, and clinical studies took the initiative to delineate the involvement of female sex per se and the female sex hormone, estrogen, in the pathogenesis of pulmonary arterial hypertension (PAH) [1, 38]. For instance, estrogen treatment shows the downregulation of expression of BMPR2, the gene that causes the expression of bone morphogenetic protein receptor II. Mutation in the BMPR2 leads to heritable pulmonary arterial hypertension in the patients [44]. Genetic variants of the cytochrome P450 and CYP1B1 increase the risk of development of pulmonary arterial hypertension in BMPR2 mutation carrier [1, 45]. This is due to the increased breakdown of estrogen into metabolites, which causes proliferation and prevents apoptosis in the vascular smooth muscle, thus narrowing the narrowing of the pulmonary vasculature. Administration of anastrozole and fulvestrant, which are estrogen receptor blockers, reversed the vascular remodeling in the BMPR2 transgenic mice [44, 46].

Clinical studies show that those women who are devoid of any cardiovascular disease are having better right ventricular ejection fraction (RVEF) compared to men [47]. This may be due to higher levels of estrogen in women. Thus, even though women are on a higher risk of getting pulmonary hypertension, and if they get the disease, their survival rate is much higher due to their better right ventricular (RV) function compared with men [48]. Research findings show that both men and post-menopausal women with pulmonary arterial hypertension have higher levels of estrogen and lower levels of dehydroepiandrosterone sulfate (DHEA-S) compared with control male and females [49]. Higher levels of estrogen are associated with shorter 6-min walk distance (6MWD), whereas a higher level of DHEA-S was linked with the lower pulmonary vascular resentence (PVR) and right atrial pressure [49].

Clinical trials were initiated to target the female sex hormone, estrogen, to manage pulmonary hypertension [50]. Findings from the small placebo-controlled randomized clinical trials (RCT) show that treatment of anastrozole reduced the circulating levels of estrogen, but no beneficial effect was observed in tricuspid annular plane systolic excursion (a marker of RV function and primary endpoint) [1]. Anastrozole significantly increased 6MWD over 12 weeks' treatment [51]. Currently, several NIH-funded trials are ongoing, targeting estrogen or androgen using fulvestrant, tamoxifen, and DHEA in the management of pulmonary artery hypertension [1, 52].

1.5.2 Genes, Epigenetics, and MicroRNAs

Research studies demonstrate that more than 70% of patients diagnosed with familial or heritable pulmonary arterial hypertension and about 20% of patients with idiopathic pulmonary arterial hypertension have heterozygous mutations in BMPR2 [1, 53]. It is almost a conclusive argument that there is a significant involvement of altered signaling of BMP in pulmonary arterial hypertension, thus targeting this pathway should be an ideal scientific acuity [53]. Multiple experimental approaches were utilized to restore BMPR2 signaling using exogenous BMPR2 delivery via gene therapy, correction of mutation through medications, improvement of trafficking of the BMPR2 to the cell membrane by chemical chaperons, inhibition of the lysosomal degradation process, and increase in BMPR2 gene expression [1].

Recent advances in the molecular and cellular biology reveal a fascinating process of the regulation of biological functions including gene expressions and pulmonary vascular physiology using small noncoding RNA molecules, termed as micro RNAs or miRNAs or miRs [54]. Dysregulation of miRs has been shown to be associated with the development and progression of PAH [54]. This suggests a potential need for a thorough investigation of the role of miRs in the pathogenesis of PAH. The possible miR therapy in the management of PAH includes the inhibitors of miR-17, miR-130/301, miR-143/145, miR-20a, and miR-10, and the mimics of miR-204, miR-424/503, and miR-96 [55]. Currently, our understanding is in infancy about the specific targets of the above miRs, and their effective delivery to the patients' body [1]. For instance, current challenges that need to be addressed include, but not limited to, the route of delivery, the mode of delivery, such as via vectors or naked oligonucleotides packaged in nanoparticles or liposomal delivery. Despite the initial hurdles, the future of the miRs therapy looks promising. miRs, via regulating the cellular gene expressions, may improve the pulmonary vascular homeostasis and thus emerge as better therapeutics tools in the management of PAH in patients [1]. One of the lead mechanisms, which cause the pulmonary vascular smooth muscle proliferation and ultimately narrowing the artery, is improper repair of the damaged DNA. This may also give rise to cancer-like phenotype and abnormal multiplication of the vascular smooth cells in PAH. Thus, DNA damage is the first step, which follows the development of PAH [56]. DNA is evident in the setting of the generation of reactive oxygen species, hypoxia, inflammation, reduced BMPR2 expression, and anorexigen drugs [56]. Consistently, the DNA damage in peripheral blood mononuclear cells, pulmonary artery smooth muscle and endothelial cells is a prior event that leads to clinical PAH [1, 56].

Downstream of DNA damages causes activation of poly (ADP-ribose) polymerase (PARP-1), which induces DNA repair process. However, research studies show overactivation of the PARP-1 pathway in clinical PAH [57]. This overactive PARP-1 signaling in PAH leads to cell dysfunction and further activation of inflammatory cell signaling response. Genetic deletion or therapeutic inhibition of PARP-1 prevents endothelial cell dysfunction, vascular remodeling, increases RV pressure and thereby attenuation of RV hypertrophy [1, 57].

In clinical studies, FK506 has been shown to significantly improve BMPR2 signaling. FK506 was tested in three advanced PAH patients who were found be resistant on the current line of treatments and were the candidates of lung transplantation [58]. FK506 improved and stabilized their conditions after 1 year of treatment. Significant improvement was observed in 6MWD, NT-ProBNP, and RV functions. Olaparib, an oral PARP-1 inhibitor, an approved drug by the FDA to treat ovarian cancer, is being investigated in an open-labeled single-arm study to investigate its effect on PVR over a 16-week duration (NCT03251872) [59]. The study is currently going on and outcomes have yet to be released [1].

1.5.3 Elastase Inhibition

Preclinical studies show a consistent finding of the disintegration of pulmonary vascular internal elastic lamina [1, 60]. This is associated with smooth muscle cell proliferation and neointima formation [60], which occurs 4 days after the monocrotaline (MCT) injection in the rats. Preclinical studies further showed that elastases, proteolytic enzymes, and target elastin can release growth factors from the extracellular matrix [60]. Treatment with the oral serine elastase inhibitor revered pulmonary vascular remodeling in MCT-exposed rats by enhancing apoptosis of smooth muscle cells. Elafin, an endogenous elastase inhibitor, is accompanied by a potent antiinflammatory activity. Elafin-overexpressed transgenic mice were found to be protected against hypoxia-induced pulmonary hypertension [46, 47]. Elafin reduced neointima formation via increasing the apoptosis in smooth muscle cells in lung in patients with PAH [61]. Elafin also demonstrated protective effects on vascular endothelium through BMPR2 and caveolin-mediated signaling mechanism [61].

Clinical studies have been initiated by the financial support of NIH to develop elafin, a potential drug to treat PAH (HL108797) [1]. These clinical investigations will assess the effectiveness, safety, and tolerability of elafin, and the effects of elafin on inflammatory markers [1].

1.5.4 Inflammation and Immunity

Inflammation induced by the generation of proinflammatory cytokines, such as IL-6, has been involved in inflammatory lung disease [62]. Mice overexpressed with IL-6 displayed an increased RV systolic pressure, hypertrophy, and severe form of occlusive angioproliferative lesions in the small distal pulmonary vessels. Besides, increased infiltration of lymphocytes was also found [48]. Deletion of IL-6 protected the mice from hypoxia-induced pulmonary hypertension [49]. Similarly, transgenic mice devoid of IL-6 receptor on the smooth muscle cells were protected against hypoxia-induced pulmonary hypertension [63]. Treatment with IL-6 receptor antagonist reversed the experiential hypertension in rats [63].

Dysregulated B-cell function, regulatory T-cell (T reg) deficiency, and pathological antibodies generation against endothelial cells are found to be associated with the pathogenesis of PAH [1, 64]. Research findings show that exposing the athymic nude rats (lacking T reg) to sugen-hypoxia resulted in increased number of B cells and generation of antiendothelial cell antibodies in pulmonary vasculature [64] and led to severe PAH [64]. Immune reconstitution using healthy T reg cells prevented accumulation of B cell and generation of antibodies against endothelial cells, resulting in attenuation of PAH [1].

Dimethyl fumarate (DMF) is NRF2 pathway-activating agent in various cell types and has been demonstrated to exert a potent antiinflammatory role in pulmonary inflammatory diseases [65]. Part of the antiinflammatory property of the DMF is through inhibition of NFkB signaling pathway. DMF is an FDA-approved medication to manage multiple sclerosis. Treatment of DMF in the sugen-hypoxia model reversed pathological hemodynamic changes, and reduced inflammation and oxidative stress [1, 65].

Clinical studies show increased levels of IL-6 in the serum of the patients diagnosed with idiopathic PAH and PAH associated with autoimmune disorders. Increased IL-6 levels are associated with increased incidents of mortality in PAH patients [66]. Increased levels of expression of IL-6 receptor have been reported in the smooth muscle cells from the patients of PAH [66].

Tocilizumab, a humanized monoclonal antibody, is approved for autoimmune disorders, such as rheumatoid arthritis [67]. Being aware of a clear role of IL-6 and its downstream singling in the pathogenesis and poor prognosis of PAH, currently, a phase II clinical study, the Therapeutic Open Label Study of Tocilizumab in the Treatment of Pulmonary Artery Hypertension (TRANSFORM-UK, NCT02676947), is underway in which Tocilizumab is administered once a month for 6 months to the patients of PAH [67]. The primary endpoints of the study are safety and change in PVR.

Based upon a potential preclinical data showing the role of Treg signaling in PAH, human trials are going on using rituximab, a chimeric monoclonal antibody against CD20, that targets B cells [1]. Rituximab has anecdotally been demonstrated to be effective with connective tissue disease (CTD)-related PAH and systemic sclerosis-associated PAH, thus requiring detailed scientific investigations of its safety and efficacy. The ASC01 study, a NIH-funded, double-blind, placebo-controlled phase II trial (NCT01086540), was initiated to evaluate the safety and efficacy of rituximab on systemic sclerosis-associated PAH and its progression. The primary endpoint is the change in PVR at 24 weeks. Secondary endpoint includes RV function measured by MRI [1].

Studies have also been initiated to target NRF-2 pathway, including the role of bardoxolone and DMF in the patients associated with systemic sclerosis-induced PAH (NCT02657356, NCT02981082) [1].

1.5.5 Mitochondrial Dysfunction

The metabolic theory of the induction of PAH is based on multiple molecular abnormalities in PAH-caused mitochondrial suppression in both pulmonary vascular cells and extrapulmonary tissue [68]. This ultimately inhibits the oxidation of the glucose metabolism and upregulation of glycolysis [68]. It is not clear yet if mitochondrial alteration is the cause or an outcome of PAH. Mitochondrial dysfunction displays an inhibition of glucose oxidation due to the abnormality at the level of the enzyme, pyruvate dehydrogenase (PVD) [68]. PVD is inhibited following the phosphorylation induced by a pyruvate dehydrogenase kinase (PDK) because of the hypoxia, inflammation, endoplasmic reticulum (ER) stress, and tyrosine kinase activation [68]. PDH inhibition leads to attenuation of apoptotic pathway, cell proliferation and inflammation—salient features of the pathogenesis of the PAH. In line with the above findings, a small molecule inhibitor, dichloroacetate (DCA), activates PDH and thereby reverses the above pathological changes in several animal models of PAH [69].

A clinical study, a 4-month, open-label trial of DCA (3–6 mg/kg b.i.d) was conducted in 20 stable WHO functional class II–III idiopathic PAH patients [70]. The results of the study showed a reduction in mPAP and PVR, and improvement in functional capacity in patients with SIRT3 and UCP2 variants that decreased PDH [70]. Based on the outcomes, further clinical studies are required to determine the drug's safety and efficacy in a large set of population.

1.5.6 Other Metabolic Pathways

Metformin, an antidiabetic drug, demonstrated the improvement in the endothelial cell function by increasing NO synthase activity and thereby reduced pulmonary artery smooth muscle cell proliferation [71]. Further studies showed that metformin also inhibits aromatase and estrogen production [72]. Metformin provided protection in MCT and hypoxia-induced PAH in rats via inhibition of smooth muscle cell proliferation [73]. Clinical studies of metformin are currently going on at Vanderbilt University for PAH (NCT01884051, NCT03617458) [1].

The mechanistic target of rapamycin complex (mTORC) pathway signals the proliferation of vascular smooth muscle cells [74]. mTORC1 and mTORC2 have been linked to PAH as their expressions are increased in pulmonary smooth muscle cells in PAH patients [75]. Studies show that mTORC2 is required for adenosine triphosphate (ATP) generation that leads to the survival of pulmonary artery smooth muscle proliferation in PAH [75]. The mTOR kinase inhibitor PP242 has a potent antiproliferative activity on mTORC2. It also induces smooth muscle cell apoptosis in small pulmonary arteries and reverses hypoxia-induced pulmonary vascular remodeling in rat model [1].

A phase I trial is initiated to investigate the effect of ABI-009, (a nanoparticle-bound rapamycin targeted to the lungs) in PAH (NCT02587325) [1].

1.5.7 Nervous System

Sympathetic nervous system activation and para-sympathetic nervous system inhibition lead to the pulmonary vascular constriction, and thereby contribute in the pathophysiology of PAH [76]. Catecholamines, upon release from sympathetic nervous system, activate α_1 receptor and thereby induce pulmonary vasoconstriction and an increase in pulmonary artery pressure [76]. However, pharmacological inhibition of α_1-receptors or activation of the parasympathetic activation causes vasorelaxation in pulmonary artery [76]. Antagonism of adrenergic receptors prevents MCT-induced pulmonary hypertension and decreases the RV size [1]. Carvedilol treatment demonstrated the improvement in survival of the animals treated with MCT [77].

Based upon animal research, several pharmacological agents targeting autonomic nervous system were investigated in clinical PAH. Small pilot studies used β-blocker such as carvedilol or bisoprolol to PAH patients [43]. The outcome of the studies showed decreased heart rate, improvement in cardiac indices and in 6MWD. A placebo-controlled crossover trial of carvedilol is current going on (NCT02507011) [1].

1.5.8 Renin-Angiotensin-Aldosterone System (RAAS)

The role of the renin-angiotensin-aldosterone system (RAAS) in the pathogenesis of PAH is recently being investigated [78]. Angiotensin II (Ang II) increases pulmonary vascular fibrosis and RV collagen deposition. Angiotensin-converting enzyme (ACE) inhibitors have a cornerstone role in the treatment of cardiovascular diseases. An increased expression of angiotensin II type 1 (AT1) receptor is observed in the pulmonary vascular of PAH patients, which may cause vasoconstriction, oxidative stress, inflammation, and smooth muscle cell proliferation. Losartan, an AT1 receptor blocker, prevented MCT-induced diseases progression, restored right ventricular (RV)-pulmonary artery (PA) coupling, and improved RV diastolic function in animals [78, 79].

Increased levels of aldosterone are reported in the blood of in animal models of PAH, as well in in some human studies [79, 80]. Administration of aldosterone receptor antagonist, spironolactone, improved RV morphology, function, and pulmonary vascular remodeling, and reduced pulmonary smooth muscle proliferation in MCT and in sugen-hypoxia rats and in hypoxia mouse model [81].

Based on the potential experimental data [82], clinical trials have been initiated and are currently going on to investigate the clinical efficacy and safety of spironolactone in patients with PAH (NCT02253394, NCT01712620, NCT01468571) [62].

1.6 Summary

Pulmonary arterial hypertension is contributing high rate of morbidity, mortality, and economic burden even in developed countries. Pulmonary vascular remodeling due to enhanced endothelial and smooth muscle cell proliferation causes the narrowing of the pulmonary artery and increases pulmonary arterial pressure. Despite recent advances in the treatment of PAH, current medications failed to halt or reverse the progression of the disease in the patients (Fig. 1.2) [6, 8]. This requires a better understanding of the disease at cellular and molecular levels. There is also a need to enhance the drug discovery process in the laboratory. Therefore, a rational drug design will yield lesser failures at preclinical and clinical stages of drug testing and may expedite the approval process of the medications to treat PAH. We hope that the medications which are currently at various stages of clinical trials will be able to change the current treatment paradigm in near future, and thus hold a promise to improve the treatment of PAH.

References

1. Spiekerkoetter E, Kawut SM, de Jesus Perez VA (2019) New and emerging therapies for pulmonary arterial hypertension. Annu Rev Med 70:45–59

2. Humbert M, Lau EM, Montani D, Jais X, Sitbon O, Simonneau G (2014) Advances in therapeutic interventions for patients with pulmonary arterial hypertension. Circulation 130 (24):2189–2208
3. Badesch DB, Champion HC, Sanchez MA, Hoeper MM, Loyd JE, Manes A et al (2009) Diagnosis and assessment of pulmonary arterial hypertension. J Am Coll Cardiol 54(1 Suppl): S55–S66
4. Thenappan T, Ormiston ML, Ryan JJ, Archer SL (2018) Pulmonary arterial hypertension: pathogenesis and clinical management. BMJ 360:j5492
5. Thenappan T, Khoruts A, Chen Y, Weir EK (2019) Can intestinal microbiota and circulating microbial products contribute to pulmonary arterial hypertension? Am J Physiol Heart Circ Physiol 317(5):H1093–HH101
6. Tsai H, Sung YK, de Jesus Perez V (2016) Recent advances in the management of pulmonary arterial hypertension. F1000Res 5:2755
7. Lau EMT, Giannoulatou E, Celermajer DS, Humbert M (2017) Epidemiology and treatment of pulmonary arterial hypertension. Nat Rev Cardiol 14(10):603–614
8. Galie N, Humbert M, Vachiery JL, Gibbs S, Lang I, Torbicki A et al (2015) 2015 ESC/ERS guidelines for the diagnosis and treatment of pulmonary hypertension: The Joint Task Force for the diagnosis and treatment of pulmonary hypertension of the European Society of Cardiology (ESC) and the European Respiratory Society (ERS): endorsed by: Association for European Paediatric and Congenital Cardiology (AEPC), International Society for Heart and Lung Transplantation (ISHLT). Eur Respir J 46(4):903–975
9. Humbert M, Sitbon O, Chaouat A, Bertocchi M, Habib G, Gressin V et al (2006) Pulmonary arterial hypertension in France: results from a national registry. Am J Respir Crit Care Med 173 (9):1023–1030
10. Mathioudakis A, Chatzimavridou-Grigoriadou V, Evangelopoulou E, Mathioudakis G (2013) Vasoactive intestinal peptide inhaled agonists: potential role in respiratory therapeutics. Hippokratia 17(1):12–16
11. Hemnes AR, Champion HC (2008) Right heart function and haemodynamics in pulmonary hypertension. Int J Clin Pract Suppl 160:11–19
12. Sysol JR, Machado RF (2018) Classification and pathophysiology of pulmonary hypertension. Continuing Cardiol Educ 4(1):2–12
13. Simonneau G, Gatzoulis MA, Adatia I, Celermajer D, Denton C, Ghofrani A et al (2013) Updated clinical classification of pulmonary hypertension. J Am Coll Cardiol 62(25 Suppl): D34–D41
14. Godbey PS, Graham JA, Presson RG Jr, Wagner WW Jr, Lloyd TC Jr (1995) Effect of capillary pressure and lung distension on capillary recruitment. J Appl Physiol (1985) 79(4):1142–1147
15. Wilkins MR, Aman J, Harbaum L, Ulrich A, Wharton J, Rhodes CJ (2018) Recent advances in pulmonary arterial hypertension. F1000Res 7. https://doi.org/10.12688/f1000research.14984.1
16. Rich JD, Rich S (2014) Clinical diagnosis of pulmonary hypertension. Circulation 130 (20):1820–1830
17. Rich S, Dantzker DR, Ayres SM, Bergofsky EH, Brundage BH, Detre KM et al (1987) Primary pulmonary hypertension. A national prospective study. Ann Intern Med 107(2):216–223
18. Soubrier F, Chung WK, Machado R, Grunig E, Aldred M, Geraci M et al (2013) Genetics and genomics of pulmonary arterial hypertension. J Am Coll Cardiol 62(25 Suppl):D13–D21
19. Deng Z, Morse JH, Slager SL, Cuervo N, Moore KJ, Venetos G et al (2000) Familial primary pulmonary hypertension (gene PPH1) is caused by mutations in the bone morphogenetic protein receptor-II gene. Am J Hum Genet 67(3):737–744
20. International PPHC, Lane KB, Machado RD, Pauciulo MW, Thomson JR, Phillips JA III et al (2000) Heterozygous germline mutations in BMPR2, encoding a TGF-beta receptor, cause familial primary pulmonary hypertension. Nat Genet 26(1):81–84
21. Abenhaim L, Moride Y, Brenot F, Rich S, Benichou J, Kurz X et al (1996) Appetite-suppressant drugs and the risk of primary pulmonary hypertension. International Primary Pulmonary Hypertension Study Group. N Engl J Med 335(9):609–616

22. Sadoughi A, Roberts KE, Preston IR, Lai GP, McCollister DH, Farber HW et al (2013) Use of selective serotonin reuptake inhibitors and outcomes in pulmonary arterial hypertension. Chest 144(2):531–541
23. Montani D, Bergot E, Gunther S, Savale L, Bergeron A, Bourdin A et al (2012) Pulmonary arterial hypertension in patients treated by dasatinib. Circulation 125(17):2128–2137
24. Melenovsky V, Kotrc M, Borlaug BA, Marek T, Kovar J, Malek I et al (2013) Relationships between right ventricular function, body composition, and prognosis in advanced heart failure. J Am Coll Cardiol 62(18):1660–1670
25. Guazzi M, Vicenzi M, Arena R, Guazzi MD (2011) Pulmonary hypertension in heart failure with preserved ejection fraction: a target of phosphodiesterase-5 inhibition in a 1-year study. Circulation 124(2):164–174
26. Seeger W, Adir Y, Barbera JA, Champion H, Coghlan JG, Cottin V et al (2013) Pulmonary hypertension in chronic lung diseases. J Am Coll Cardiol 62(25 Suppl):D109–D116
27. Kim NH, Delcroix M, Jenkins DP, Channick R, Dartevelle P, Jansa P et al (2013) Chronic thromboembolic pulmonary hypertension. J Am Coll Cardiol 62(25 Suppl):D92–D99
28. Mahmud E, Madani MM, Kim NH, Poch D, Ang L, Behnamfar O et al (2018) Chronic thromboembolic pulmonary hypertension: evolving therapeutic approaches for operable and inoperable disease. J Am Coll Cardiol 71(21):2468–2486
29. Gordeuk VR, Castro OL, Machado RF (2016) Pathophysiology and treatment of pulmonary hypertension in sickle cell disease. Blood 127(7):820–828
30. Farber HW, Loscalzo J (2004) Pulmonary arterial hypertension. N Engl J Med 351 (16):1655–1665
31. Gerber JG, Voelkel N, Nies AS, McMurtry IF, Reeves JT (1980) Moderation of hypoxic vasoconstriction by infused arachidonic acid: role of PGI2. J Appl Physiol Respir Environ Exerc Physiol 49(1):107–112
32. Christman BW, McPherson CD, Newman JH, King GA, Bernard GR, Groves BM et al (1992) An imbalance between the excretion of thromboxane and prostacyclin metabolites in pulmonary hypertension. N Engl J Med 327(2):70–75
33. Allen SW, Chatfield BA, Koppenhafer SA, Schaffer MS, Wolfe RR, Abman SH (1993) Circulating immunoreactive endothelin-1 in children with pulmonary hypertension. Association with acute hypoxic pulmonary vasoreactivity. Am Rev Respir Dis 148(2):519–522
34. Komai H, Adatia IT, Elliott MJ, de Leval MR, Haworth SG (1993) Increased plasma levels of endothelin-1 after cardiopulmonary bypass in patients with pulmonary hypertension and congenital heart disease. J Thorac Cardiovasc Surg 106(3):473–478
35. Giaid A, Saleh D (1995) Reduced expression of endothelial nitric oxide synthase in the lungs of patients with pulmonary hypertension. N Engl J Med 333(4):214–221
36. Xue C, Johns RA (1995) Endothelial nitric oxide synthase in the lungs of patients with pulmonary hypertension. N Engl J Med 333(24):1642–1644
37. Jiao YR, Wang W, Lei PC, Jia HP, Dong J, Gou YQ et al (2019) 5-HTT, BMPR2, EDN1, ENG, KCNA5 gene polymorphisms and susceptibility to pulmonary arterial hypertension: a meta-analysis. Gene 680:34–42
38. Marcos E, Fadel E, Sanchez O, Humbert M, Dartevelle P, Simonneau G et al (2004) Serotonin-induced smooth muscle hyperplasia in various forms of human pulmonary hypertension. Circ Res 94(9):1263–1270
39. Baliga RS, Macallister RJ, Hobbs AJ (2013) Vasoactive peptides and the pathogenesis of pulmonary hypertension: role and potential therapeutic application. Handb Exp Pharmacol 218:477–511
40. Voelkel NF, Gomez-Arroyo J (2014) The role of vascular endothelial growth factor in pulmonary arterial hypertension. The angiogenesis paradox. Am J Respir Cell Mol Biol 51 (4):474–484
41. Schermuly RT, Ghofrani HA, Wilkins MR, Grimminger F (2011) Mechanisms of disease: pulmonary arterial hypertension. Nat Rev Cardiol 8(8):443–455

42. Guignabert C, Tu L, Girerd B, Ricard N, Huertas A, Montani D et al (2015) New molecular targets of pulmonary vascular remodeling in pulmonary arterial hypertension: importance of endothelial communication. Chest 147(2):529–537
43. da Silva Goncalves Bos D, Van Der Bruggen CEE, Kurakula K, Sun XQ, Casali KR, Casali AG et al (2018) Contribution of impaired parasympathetic activity to right ventricular dysfunction and pulmonary vascular remodeling in pulmonary arterial hypertension. Circulation 137 (9):910–924
44. Lahm T, Tuder RM, Petrache I (2014) Progress in solving the sex hormone paradox in pulmonary hypertension. Am J Physiol Lung Cell Mol Physiol 307(1):L7–L26
45. Austin ED, Hamid R, Hemnes AR, Loyd JE, Blackwell T, Yu C et al (2012) BMPR2 expression is suppressed by signaling through the estrogen receptor. Biol Sex Differ 3(1):6
46. Chen X, Austin ED, Talati M, Fessel JP, Farber-Eger EH, Brittain EL et al (2017) Oestrogen inhibition reverses pulmonary arterial hypertension and associated metabolic defects. Eur Respir J 50(2):1602337
47. Kawut SM, Lima JA, Barr RG, Chahal H, Jain A, Tandri H et al (2011) Sex and race differences in right ventricular structure and function: the multi-ethnic study of atherosclerosis-right ventricle study. Circulation 123(22):2542–2551
48. Jacobs W, van de Veerdonk MC, Trip P, de Man F, Heymans MW, Marcus JT et al (2014) The right ventricle explains sex differences in survival in idiopathic pulmonary arterial hypertension. Chest 145(6):1230–1236
49. Hemnes AR, Maynard KB, Champion HC, Gleaves L, Penner N, West J et al (2012) Testosterone negatively regulates right ventricular load stress responses in mice. Pulm Circ 2(3):352–358
50. Austin ED, Cogan JD, West JD, Hedges LK, Hamid R, Dawson EP et al (2009) Alterations in oestrogen metabolism: implications for higher penetrance of familial pulmonary arterial hypertension in females. Eur Respir J 34(5):1093–1099
51. Kawut SM, Archer-Chicko CL, DeMichele A, Fritz JS, Klinger JR, Ky B et al (2017) Anastrozole in pulmonary arterial hypertension. A randomized, double-blind, placebo-controlled trial. Am J Respir Crit Care Med 195(3):360–368
52. Baird GL, Archer-Chicko C, Barr RG, Bluemke DA, Foderaro AE, Fritz JS et al (2018) Lower DHEA-S levels predict disease and worse outcomes in post-menopausal women with idiopathic, connective tissue disease- and congenital heart disease-associated pulmonary arterial hypertension. Eur Respir J 51(6):1800467
53. Orriols M, Gomez-Puerto MC, Ten Dijke P (2017) BMP type II receptor as a therapeutic target in pulmonary arterial hypertension. Cell Mol Life Sci 74(16):2979–2995
54. Boucherat O, Bonnet S (2016) MicroRNA signature of end-stage idiopathic pulmonary arterial hypertension: clinical correlations and regulation of WNT signaling. J Mol Med (Berl) 94 (8):849–851
55. Chun HJ, Bonnet S, Chan SY (2017) Translational advances in the field of pulmonary hypertension. Translating microRNA biology in pulmonary hypertension. It will take more than "miR" words. Am J Respir Crit Care Med 195(2):167–178
56. Ranchoux B, Meloche J, Paulin R, Boucherat O, Provencher S, Bonnet S (2016) DNA damage and pulmonary hypertension. Int J Mol Sci 17(6)
57. Kaur G, Singh N, Lingeshwar P, Siddiqui HH, Hanif K (2015) Poly (ADP-ribose) polymerase-1: an emerging target in right ventricle dysfunction associated with pulmonary hypertension. Pulm Pharmacol Ther 30:66–79
58. Lallouet M, Sornin G (1985) [Craniomandibular joint dysfunction. Report of a clinical case]. Inf Dent 67(36):3811–3812
59. Spiekerkoetter E, Sung YK, Sudheendra D, Scott V, Del Rosario P, Bill M et al (2017) Randomised placebo-controlled safety and tolerability trial of FK506 (tacrolimus) for pulmonary arterial hypertension. Eur Respir J 50(3)
60. Maruyama K, Ye CL, Woo M, Venkatacharya H, Lines LD, Silver MM et al (1991) Chronic hypoxic pulmonary hypertension in rats and increased elastolytic activity. Am J Phys 261(6 Pt 2):H1716–H1726

61. Zaidi SH, You XM, Ciura S, Husain M, Rabinovitch M (2002) Overexpression of the serine elastase inhibitor elafin protects transgenic mice from hypoxic pulmonary hypertension. Circulation 105(4):516–521
62. Steiner MK, Syrkina OL, Kolliputi N, Mark EJ, Hales CA, Waxman AB (2009) Interleukin-6 overexpression induces pulmonary hypertension. Circ Res 104(2):236–44, 28p following 44
63. Tamura Y, Phan C, Tu L, Le Hiress M, Thuillet R, Jutant EM et al (2018) Ectopic upregulation of membrane-bound IL6R drives vascular remodeling in pulmonary arterial hypertension. J Clin Invest 128(5):1956–1970
64. Taraseviciene-Stewart L, Nicolls MR, Kraskauskas D, Scerbavicius R, Burns N, Cool C et al (2007) Absence of T cells confers increased pulmonary arterial hypertension and vascular remodeling. Am J Respir Crit Care Med 175(12):1280–1289
65. Grzegorzewska AP, Seta F, Han R, Czajka CA, Makino K, Stawski L et al (2017) Dimethyl fumarate ameliorates pulmonary arterial hypertension and lung fibrosis by targeting multiple pathways. Sci Rep 7:41605
66. Soon E, Holmes AM, Treacy CM, Doughty NJ, Southgate L, Machado RD et al (2010) Elevated levels of inflammatory cytokines predict survival in idiopathic and familial pulmonary arterial hypertension. Circulation 122(9):920–927
67. Hernandez-Sanchez J, Harlow L, Church C, Gaine S, Knightbridge E, Bunclark K et al (2018) Clinical trial protocol for TRANSFORM-UK: a therapeutic open-label study of tocilizumab in the treatment of pulmonary arterial hypertension. Pulm Circ 8(1):2045893217735820
68. Paulin R, Michelakis ED (2014) The metabolic theory of pulmonary arterial hypertension. Circ Res 115(1):148–164
69. McMurtry MS, Bonnet S, Wu X, Dyck JR, Haromy A, Hashimoto K et al (2004) Dichloroacetate prevents and reverses pulmonary hypertension by inducing pulmonary artery smooth muscle cell apoptosis. Circ Res 95(8):830–840
70. Michelakis ED, Gurtu V, Webster L, Barnes G, Watson G, Howard L et al (2017) Inhibition of pyruvate dehydrogenase kinase improves pulmonary arterial hypertension in genetically susceptible patients. Sci Transl Med 9(413)
71. Sartoretto JL, Melo GA, Carvalho MH, Nigro D, Passaglia RT, Scavone C et al (2005) Metformin treatment restores the altered microvascular reactivity in neonatal streptozotocin-induced diabetic rats increasing NOS activity, but not NOS expression. Life Sci 77 (21):2676–2689
72. Dean A, Nilsen M, Loughlin L, Salt IP, MacLean MR (2016) Metformin reverses development of pulmonary hypertension via aromatase inhibition. Hypertension 68(2):446–454
73. Agard C, Rolli-Derkinderen M, Dumas-de-La-Roque E, Rio M, Sagan C, Savineau JP et al (2009) Protective role of the antidiabetic drug metformin against chronic experimental pulmonary hypertension. Br J Pharmacol 158(5):1285–1294
74. Pena A, Kobir A, Goncharov D, Goda A, Kudryashova TV, Ray A et al (2017) Pharmacological inhibition of mTOR kinase reverses right ventricle remodeling and improves right ventricle structure and function in rats. Am J Respir Cell Mol Biol 57(5):615–625
75. Goncharov DA, Kudryashova TV, Ziai H, Ihida-Stansbury K, DeLisser H, Krymskaya VP et al (2014) Mammalian target of rapamycin complex 2 (mTORC2) coordinates pulmonary artery smooth muscle cell metabolism, proliferation, and survival in pulmonary arterial hypertension. Circulation 129(8):864–874
76. Vaillancourt M, Chia P, Sarji S, Nguyen J, Hoftman N, Ruffenach G et al (2017) Autonomic nervous system involvement in pulmonary arterial hypertension. Respir Res 18(1):201
77. Drake JI, Gomez-Arroyo J, Dumur CI, Kraskauskas D, Natarajan R, Bogaard HJ et al (2013) Chronic carvedilol treatment partially reverses the right ventricular failure transcriptional profile in experimental pulmonary hypertension. Physiol Genomics 45(12):449–461
78. de Man FS, Tu L, Handoko ML, Rain S, Ruiter G, Francois C et al (2012) Dysregulated renin-angiotensin-aldosterone system contributes to pulmonary arterial hypertension. Am J Respir Crit Care Med 186(8):780–789

79. Shenoy V, Kwon KC, Rathinasababapathy A, Lin S, Jin G, Song C et al (2014) Oral delivery of Angiotensin-converting enzyme 2 and Angiotensin-(1-7) bioencapsulated in plant cells attenuates pulmonary hypertension. Hypertension 64(6):1248–1259
80. Maron BA, Opotowsky AR, Landzberg MJ, Loscalzo J, Waxman AB, Leopold JA (2013) Plasma aldosterone levels are elevated in patients with pulmonary arterial hypertension in the absence of left ventricular heart failure: a pilot study. Eur J Heart Fail 15(3):277–283
81. Maron BA, Oldham WM, Chan SY, Vargas SO, Arons E, Zhang YY et al (2014) Upregulation of steroidogenic acute regulatory protein by hypoxia stimulates aldosterone synthesis in pulmonary artery endothelial cells to promote pulmonary vascular fibrosis. Circulation 130 (2):168–179
82. Hemnes AR, Rathinasababapathy A, Austin EA, Brittain EL, Carrier EJ, Chen X et al (2018) A potential therapeutic role for angiotensin-converting enzyme 2 in human pulmonary arterial hypertension. Eur Respir J 51(6)

Asthma: Pathophysiology, Current Status, and Therapeutics

2

Javeed Ahmad Bhat, Nawab John Dar, and Wajid Waheed Bhat

Abstract

Asthma is a chronic disorder of the airways characterized by variable and recurring airway inflammation, bronchial hyperresponsiveness, bronchoconstriction, vasodilatation, airway edema, and activation of sensory nerve endings. It is a serious health problem globally affecting 334 million people across all the age groups imposing a substantial burden on patient's quality of life, family, and community. Patients with asthma are often at the risk of acute exacerbations, if the symptoms are not managed properly, and it needs to be customized based on the level of symptom control, phenotypic characteristics, effectiveness of available medications, safety, cost-effectiveness, etc. Since the underlying pathophysiological mechanisms and symptoms of the disease are complicated, there is a dire need to understand the pathology of the disease for better management of symptoms and development of novel therapeutic approaches. Here, we have presented a comprehensive review of the disease, its causes, epidemiology, pathophysiology, current drug treatments, and latest recommendations from Global Initiative for Asthma for the management of asthma.

J. A. Bhat
Department of Biochemistry and Biophysics, University of Rochester Medical Center, Rochester, NY, USA

N. J. Dar (✉)
Department of Cell Systems and Anatomy, School of Medicine, UT Health, San Antonio, TX, USA
e-mail: darn@uthscsa.edu

W. W. Bhat
Department of Biochemistry and Molecular Biology, Michigan State University, East Lansing, MI, USA

S. Rayees et al. (eds.), *Chronic Lung Diseases*,
https://doi.org/10.1007/978-981-15-3734-9_2

Keywords

Asthma · Airway inflammation · Bronchial hyperresponsiveness · Bronchoconstriction · Vasodilatation · Airway edema · Epidemiology · Pathophysiology · GINA

2.1 Introduction

Asthma is an obstructive pulmonary disorder with exacerbations characterized by symptoms of shortness of breath, cough, chest tightness, and/or wheezing due to restricted transportation of air to and from lungs. The symptoms of disease often occur in periodic attacks due to congestion in chest, breathlessness, severe bronchial response, inflammation, wheezing, and coughing [1–3]. Asthma occurs both in adults and in children. In children, onset of asthma occurs as early as 5 years. Asthma attacks range from mild to severe and usually occur when symptoms are at peak. In some cases, severe asthma attacks prevent oxygen from reaching lungs, which in turn may hinder with oxygenation of blood, flowing to vital organs as well. Initially during asthma attack, enough air is supplied to lungs with very limited exchange of carbon dioxide, and if it prolongs, there may be buildup of poisonous carbon dioxide which may further hinder in oxygenation of bloodstream, and such attacks need immediate medical attention. Though there is no known remedy for asthma, yet it can be controlled by proper medical care and by avoiding factors like environmental risks and other factors which otherwise may trigger severe attacks [4]. Though no specific classification of asthma has been given, yet depending upon different factors like age, gender, and environment, asthma has been broadly divided into following types.

2.1.1 Childhood Asthma

Children are likely to suffer from intermittent form of asthma, which may be followed by severe attacks. Typically, children suffer mainly due to environmental risk factors which otherwise are triggering elements for asthma. Secondhand smoke has been found to be main cause for severe asthma attacks of children, and according to American Lung Association, somewhere in between 400,000 and one million children suffer due to secondhand smoke. Moreover, according to the Centers for Disease Control and Prevention (CDC), it has been found that children have been admitted in emergency more often than adults. It has been also found that mild asthma may be treated during early childhood; however, risk factor remains intact as conditions may recur later on especially if symptoms were found to be moderate or severe [5–7].

2.1.2 Adult-Onset Asthma

Asthma can begin at any age, but usually, adult asthma is associated with severe attacks and often persists, which then requires daily management. Interestingly, it has been found that males get more affected in childhood, whereas role is reversed after the age of 20. Among many risk factors, obesity has been found to be main cause for asthma of women, though other factors cannot be ruled out. Although, in early years, asthma is manageable with Medicare, it has been found to be more lethal after age 65 where maximum deaths have been recorded due to asthma [8–14].

2.1.3 Occupational Asthma

This is kind of asthma where your environment will play a pivotal role and is directly related to your surroundings like job, home, or other occasional company. Symptoms may become active after attending particular environment, especially the places like industries, laboratory, hospitals, or other such places which have been found to be associated with occupational asthma [15].

2.1.4 Difficult-to-Control and Severe Asthma

In this kind of asthma, the symptoms reach to the level where it is difficult to control the severe attacks with the current medication, though symptoms could be controlled to some extent. These types of asthmatic patients often feel difficulty in breathing and have congestion. There is a need of new medication in this direction though there has been a lot of improvement in yesteryears with new medications like eosinophilic asthma which otherwise do not link to any allergic reactions.

2.1.5 Seasonal Asthma

This is a kind of asthma where people otherwise have asthma throughout the year but feel symptoms only in response to allergens which are season-dependent like pollen in hay fever or cold air in winter season.

2.2 Causes

In the recent past, it has been a matter of debate, whether genetic, epigenetic, or environmental factors alone or together are responsible for development of asthma. Among many, following are few primary reasons for development of asthma.

2.2.1 Genetics

There is a school of thought which believes that asthma runs through families from generation to generation. It has been found that identical twins are more likely to have same asthma condition as compared to nonidentical twins. Furthermore, studies have suggested that if one parent is having asthma, child is 25% susceptible, whereas in case of both parents, susceptibility increases to 50%, which shows, in fact, asthma is genetic. Though there are no solid conclusions for such studies, yet as how these effects differ with different environments puts epigenetic study of asthma on the heart of further research [16–18].

2.2.2 Allergies

Allergies are thought to be one of the main causes for asthma, as there has been strong correlation between two. In one of many studies, in 2013, *Annals of Asthma, Allergy, and Immunology* suggested that over 65% of adults with asthma above age of 55 years was found to be allergic as well, which may well go up to 75% between 20 and 40 years. Some of the common sources of allergens are animal proteins, dust, insects like cockroaches, fungi, cotton, and cooking.

2.2.3 Smoking Tobacco

There are endless reports from decades where smoking tobacco has been shown directly proportional to asthma, and smoking has been established as a confirmed risk factor for asthma. Smoking has been found to directly involve with cough, wheezing, and other respiratory infections, which may lead to death as well. Prenatal exposure to smoke has been found severe effect on children in relation to development of asthma symptoms. It has been found that children whose parents smoke are more prone to asthma development. Smoking worsens conditions in asthma by coughing, breathlessness, and formation of extra mucus, thus making asthma patient susceptible to other infections as well. Asthma severity has been found to be realty reduced upon less exposure to tobacco smoke [19–22].

2.2.4 Environmental Factors

Air pollution also plays a pivotal role in asthma formation though effect is not as prominent as tobacco smoke. Air pollution could be found both in and out of the home. Some of the main risk factors of air pollution indoor are cooking on indoor open fire, mold or fumes from paints, and household cleaners, and outdoor air pollution includes suspension particles or sulfur dioxide, nitrogen dioxide, pollen, ozone, cold temperature, high humidity, and wood fires among many others. All these risk factors lead to different symptoms of asthma like coughing, breathlessness, and congestion. Sometimes, heavy air pollution contributes to greater recurrence of asthma symptoms due to the emission of poisonous gases like sulfur dioxide, nitrogen dioxide, and ozone.

2.2.5 Obesity

According to American Academy of Asthma, Allergies, and Immunology, obesity is considered to be not so prominent risk factor for asthma, yet there are some studies which suggest otherwise. There had been evidences where it has been seen that the diets which were recommended to reduce cardiovascular diseases and cancers were found to reduce asthma as well. It has been found that fast food increases the risk of asthma, and hence, there is a prominent school of thought who believe obesity and asthma are very much linked with each other [23–25].

2.2.6 Pregnancy

Smoking during pregnancy makes child prone to various medical and physical conditions among which growth of baby, complication during labor and delivery, weight of baby, and child becoming more prone to asthma are among few of many [26–29].

2.2.7 The Menstrual Cycle

Premenstrual asthma (PMA) has been found to lead to acute symptoms due to sensitivity to aspirin during menstrual cycle. It has been found that hormones like luteinizing hormone (LH) and follicle-stimulating hormone (FSH), regulating menstrual cycle, influence the immune activity, and this can lead to hypersensitivity of airways.

2.2.8 Atopy

When the allergic hypersensitivity causes allergic reactions in different body parts without being in contact with allergens such as hay fever and allergic conjunctivitis, it is known as atopy. Immunoglobulin (IgE) antibodies are usually produced in more numbers than in response to usually common allergens. Atopic asthma is a most common type, where due to atopy in response to environmental allergens overproduction of (IgE) antibodies occurs, which triggers asthmatic attacks [25].

2.3 Epidemiology/Morbidity (Global Status)

Asthma is comprehensively substantial noncommunicable chronic disease with major public health consequences for both children and adults, including high morbidity and mortality in severe cases affecting approximately 334 million people worldwide. The ethnicity and socioeconomic status has an influence on the prevalence, morbidity, and mortality of the disease in the United States and various countries throughout the world [30, 31]. Reports have shown that people with asthma are more susceptible to infections and noncommunicable chronic comorbidities that result in worsening the condition of the patients with asthma. It has been reported to put a huge burden at the societal, financial, and healthcare levels of multiple nations [32–34]. Defining the global incidence and prevalence of asthma with accuracy is a challenging task because the diagnosis is based on survey responses to questions about relatively nonspecific symptoms which are open to subjective interpretation [35–37]. The International Study of Asthma and Allergy in Childhood has a validated questionnaire, which was used in 56 countries among children aged 6–14 years and is one of the frequently used tools for identifying asthma in children [37, 38]. In the same way, a validated instrument for adults is based on the European Community Respiratory Health Survey questionnaire [35, 37]. In the United States, the National Health Interview Survey (NHIS) conducted by the Centers for Disease Control and Prevention (CDC) routinely collects data about prevalence using self-reported symptoms (such as history of wheezing) using validated measures [39]. Globally, asthma is ranked 16th among the leading causes of years lived with disability and 28th among the leading causes of burden of disease, as measured by disability-adjusted life years [40]. Currently, in the United States, the prevalence of asthma among adults is approximately 7.6%, but rates vary intensely among different ethnic groups. The reported prevalence is 9.1% among black non-Hispanics and 13.6% among Puerto Ricans but only approximately 5% for Mexican and Asians [41, 42]. Globally, most data available on ethnic-related differences in asthma prevalence come either from the United Kingdom (UK) or from Canada. Although similar rates of asthma have been reported, however, they found increased risk for admissions, among black and South Asian populations in the UK. Further, the reports have found that Chinese children born in Canada had higher rates of asthma than those who were born in China [43–45]. A report from World Health Organization (WHO) has revealed a list of countries with the highest prevalence of clinical asthma, which include the percentage as Australia (21.5%), Sweden (20.2%), UK (18.2%), the Netherlands (15.3%), and Brazil (13.0%); however, the United States and Canada were excluded. The lowest rates were observed in Vietnam (1.0%), Bosnia–Herzegovina (1.4%), and China (1.4%) [46]. The lower asthma prevalence rates in Asia and Africa are believed to be linked with environmental and lifestyle causes than genetic differences [47]. While comparing the mortality rates from chronic diseases, the mortality rate for the asthma accounts for less than 1% of deaths globally. However, given the high prevalence worldwide, asthma is still responsible for 250,000 potentially preventable deaths annually [37, 48–50]. In the United States, mortality is highest among African

Americans and Puerto Ricans and individuals of Cuban descent. According to the WHO mortality database, South Africa had the highest age-standardized asthma mortality among the low- and middle-income countries, while the Netherlands had the lowest among the high-income countries [30, 51].

2.4 Pathophysiology of Asthma

Asthma is a highly intricate condition in which the clinical signs are caused due to obstruction of the conducting airways of lung. The pathophysiology of the disease is largely undefined. It is characterized by airway hyperresponsiveness, mucus hyperproduction, reversible air flow obstruction, and airway wall remodeling [52]. Although there have been huge improvements in therapeutic interventions, asthma still remains a challenge worldwide [53]. It is typically believed as distinct Th2 disease, with augmented IgE levels and eosinophilic inflammation in the airway [54]. Clinically, patients with poor asthma control have difficulties with daily life activities, exercise, and sleep repeatedly. Moreover, frequent recurrent exacerbations are further compromising patient quality of life in these patients [55].

2.4.1 Airway Inflammation and Remodeling

Numerous preclinical and clinical studies have shown that airway inflammation plays a key role in disease pathophysiology. Chronic airway inflammation induced by the action of mediators from inflammatory cells is characterized over years in asthma. The inflammatory cascade has shown to have intense magnitudes on the mechanics of airway narrowing in asthma, thus contributing toward the severity and progression of the disease [54]. Under normal physiological conditions, the human airway has shown to maintain an adequate balance between immune cells, the epithelium, and the host immune response. However, this balance has been shown to be altered during airway inflammation in asthma orchestrating *via* complex interplay between multiple effectors and targets. It has been observed that patients who die of this disease have inflamed airways subverted with inflammatory cells, primarily T lymphocytes and eosinophils [56]. Epithelium in airway is shedding in patches perpetually signifying the presence of epithelial cells in the airway lumen. The inflammation in asthmatic airways has demonstrated to extend to the terminal bronchioles besides trachea and bronchi [57]. Moreover, studies have suggested the presence of inflammatory cells in the parenchyma using transbronchial biopsies [58]. Although the association between inflammation and clinical symptoms of asthma is not clear, there is a possible link between the inflammation and airway hyperresponsiveness. The augmented airway responsiveness in asthma is a remarkable physiological abnormality demonstrated even if the airway function is found to be normal. It may be due to aberrant behavior of airway smooth muscle, increased release of mediators, edema, and irreversible airway smooth-muscle (ASM) thickening. Furthermore, airway sensory nerves may also lead to symptoms like cough and chest tightness [59]. Furthermore, increased airway wall thickness contributes to airway narrowing during (ASM) contraction *via* symmetrical effects [60, 61]. Mucosal layer thickness and the airway smooth muscle stimulate the surge in airway resistance for any given volume of airway smooth-muscle shortening. Air wall present on the outer side of the airway smooth muscle has shown to decrease the elastic pull of the attached lung, thus resulting in lowering the force against which airway smooth muscle has to shorten [62]. Cellular hyperplasia and hypertrophy in airway smooth muscle possibly increase force generation albeit the contractile processes remain normal. Conversely, airway smooth muscles are greatly plastic, indicating that it can change its contractile phenotype as soon as exposed to inflammatory mediators, tenacious contraction, and altered length, therefore contributing toward airway hyperresponsiveness [63–65]. The inflammation-induced airway injury to the epithelium is repaired *via* injury–repair cycle by recruiting different cell types which contribute toward airway remodeling. Airway segments function *via* an integrated system rather in isolation. They are unified into the moving, branching system of airways working in parallel and in series. Remodeling and inflammation of airways is possibly distributed irregularly over this branching system in patients with severe asthma [66]. Postmortem reports from patients using lung resection and transbronchial biopsies have demonstrated eosinophilic, neutrophilic, and lymphocytic inflammation and remodeling in the peripheral airways extending to the adventitia and lung as seen in the large airways [67–69]. Remodeling of the ASM in the small airways bears a resemblance to ASM remodeling in the large airways. It has been found that inflammation in the small airways may possibly disrupt the adjacent adventitial attachments in fatal asthma and diminish elastic recoil pressure, pronounced in long-standing asthma and during asthma exacerbations [70, 71]. There has been a growing interest in the mechanism of airway wall remodeling in asthma comprehending that airway inflammation alone is inadequate to describe the progression or chronicity of asthma [72]. The airway remodeling could be considered in relation to extracellular matrix deposition. Reports have suggested that the injured airway epithelium acts as a continuous stimulus for airway remodeling [72]. The remodeling is expected to have slight influence on baseline respiratory mechanics. The accumulation of extracellular matrix is reported to have physiological effects that may result in an exaggerated degree of narrowing for a given amount of airway smooth-muscle (ASM) contraction [54]. Remodeling involves degradation and repair of extracellular matrix (ECM) and proliferation of fibroblasts and myofibroblasts. The action of matrix metalloproteinases on ECM releases pro-inflammatory factors and surge neovascularization. Elastin fragments are pro-inflammatory and pro-proliferative stimulating matrix degradation via stimulating matrix metalloproteinase release [73]. Among the pathological processes that are linked with bronchial inflammation and remodeling in asthma, airway epithelium has revealed to play a key role. It has shown to represent beyond a protective blockade against external insults, as it actively secretes pro-inflammatory mediators, that is, cytokines such as IL-8 and thymic stromal lymphopoietin (TSLP) and leukotrienes which in turn augment the primary inflammation by recruiting and activating neutrophils in the early phase and eosinophils and lymphocytes during the late response [74].

2.4.2 Airway Epithelium

Airway inflammation has shown to damage the epithelium and leads to epithelial wall shedding, which is one of the distinguishing features of asthma. However, these epithelial cells are gradually repaired *via* injury–repair cycle. Epithelium injury has shown to escalate epidermal growth factor (EGF) receptor expression persistently at the site of injury, which may result the epithelium to be locked in a repair phenotype [75].

The airway epithelium has shown to control inflammatory, immune, and regenerative responses toward pollutants, chemical sensitizers, allergens, and viruses significantly that subsidize to asthma pathogenesis. Epithelial cells have demonstrated pattern recognition receptors that detect environmental stimuli and secrete endogenous detrimental signals, thereby activating dendritic cells and bridging innate and adaptive immunity [76]. The damage in epithelial wall has demonstrated to contribute toward the progression of AHR in numerous ways including loss in enzyme activity that degrades inflammatory mediators (e.g., neutral endopeptidase) and sensory nerve exposure leading to reflex neural effects [77]. Epithelial cells that shed from the airway wall may be found in bunches in the BAL fluid or sputum (Creola bodies) of asthmatics, suggesting loss of attachment to the basal layer or basement membrane. The damaged epithelium may contribute to AHR in numerous ways such as loss of its barrier function to allow penetration of allergens and irritants, enzymes (endopeptidases), relaxant factors, surfactant function, and edema and swelling [78]. Reports have shown that during injury–repair cycle, epithelial cells produce some pro-fibrotic factors, including transforming growth factor-β, fibroblast growth factor, and endothelin, regulating fibroblast and myofibroblast to release elastic fiber, collagen, proteoglycan, and glycoprotein which in turn induce airway wall thickening [79].

2.4.3 Airway Smooth Muscle

Airway smooth muscle (ASM) plays a fundamental role in the pathophysiology of asthma. It is responsible for acute bronchoconstriction, which is believed to be stimulated by constrictor hyperresponsiveness, impaired relaxation, and length adaptation. ASM further contributes to airway remodeling and inflammation in asthma [80]. Increased ASM mass has been recognized as a hallmark of asthma, and its adequate presence is predominantly found in fatal [81] or severe cases [82]. Airway structural alterations are selectively associated with severe asthma [83]. The mechanisms behind such excess accumulation are still debatable. Both increased ASM cell size (hypertrophy) and cell number (hyperplasia) have been demonstrated with hypertrophy being prime in some subjects and hyperplasia characteristic of others. Reports using single ASM cells and on ASM-impregnated gel cultures have shown that asthmatic ASM is intrinsically hypercontractile. Several elements of the ASM contraction apparatus in asthmatics and in animal models of asthma have been found to be different from nonasthmatics. These differences include some regulatory contractile proteins and also some components of both the calcium-dependent and calcium-independent contraction signaling pathways [84]. There is evidence that ASM plays a pivotal role in the airway inflammation characteristic of asthma as well. It has shown to release and express several molecular signals that contribute to bronchial inflammation and have become targets of novel therapeutic strategies [85]. Numerous studies have suggested that the airway smooth muscle in asthma is phenotypically different from normal airway smooth muscle and that these changes reflect the impact of the inflammatory asthmatic airway microenvironment on smooth muscle [86]. Airway smooth muscle is not only influenced by the inflammatory mediators and cytokines where it is occupied [87], but recent reports have shown that airway smooth muscle modulates the remodeling process by secreting multiple cytokines, growth factors, or matrix proteins and by expressing cell adhesion molecules and other potential molecules [85] like increased numbers of mast cells that have been identified in airway smooth muscle of patients with asthma [88].

2.4.4 Airway Mucus Hypersecretion

Airway mucus hypersecretion is regarded as a crucial pathophysiological feature in many patients with asthma, chronic obstructive pulmonary disease (COPD), and cystic fibrosis [89]. Reports have demonstrated that among the patients with asthma, mucus hypersecretion had more dyspnea, poorer asthma control and quality of life, and further on suffered more exacerbations. Moreover, these patients have demonstrated anosmia associated with chronic rhinosinusitis and nasal polyposis more frequently [90]. Long back in 1880s, autopsy studies have revealed that widespread airway mucus plugging is a principal cause of death from asthma [46]. These findings were significantly confirmed in numerous studies [91]. Quantitative studies have found that around 98% of airways were occluded to some extent by mucus in fatal asthma [92]. However, the contribution of mucus hypersecretion to airflow obstruction in nonfatal asthma relative to other contributors to airway closure such as extravagated plasma and to airway narrowing from smooth-muscle contraction and wall thickening remains to be determined [93]. Studies using Foxa2 knockout mice have shown increase in baseline airway and lung tissue resistance with spontaneous MUC5AC overproduction, suggesting a substantial role for mucus [94]. There is evidence for hyperplasia of submucosal glands which are confined to large airways and of increased numbers of epithelial goblet cells in patients with asthma, especially those with severe asthma [95]. Numerous reports have revealed that MUC5AC (mucin gene) is induced by complement factor C3a, tumor necrosis factor (TNF)-α NO, EGF family ligands, or neutrophil elastase [96–99].

2.5 Cell Types Involved in Asthma

Th2 lymphocyte secreting type 2 cytokines are recognized to mediate pathophysiology of asthma. Nonetheless, there are other cell types that are majorly involved, including mast cells eosinophils, $CD4^+$ T-lymphocytes, dendritic cells, and macrophages [100]. In asthma patients, eosinophils in the airways are recruited through a chemical gradient due to the release of chemotactic agents and indicate a sustained survival, persuading epithelial injury and remodeling by releasing eosinophilic toxic agents. Increased recruitment of lymphocytes and decreased cell apoptosis may result in accumulation of T lymphocytes within the airways [101]. This increase in the recruitment is possibly stimulated due to the release of lymphokines including TSLP [102]. The structural and immune cells of the airways have shown to express TSLP at the allergen entry playing a key role in switching allergy-mediated inflammation as it regulates and pushes Th2 responses [103]. With the development of the asthma in different phases like induction phase, early-phase, and the late-phase asthmatic reaction, different cell types are known to play diverse roles at all the three stages. Antigen-presenting cells are the most active at the induction phase, while as mast cells at the early and eosinophils, neutrophils, and other cell types are found to play vital role in the late phases of the diseases [104].

2.5.1 Dendritic Cells

Dendritic cells (DCs) are principal antigen-presenting cells interacting with T cells for the initiation of proliferative processes among Th1 or Th2 cell types. During the initial allergic reactions when a foreign substance reaches to the upper airways, it may be retained on the epithelium of trachea, bronchi, or alveoli. At this point, it could possibly be cleared by mucociliary transport or it would be taken up by sentinel cells. Here, dendritic cells (DCs) are the most essential sentinel cells that play a role in antigen presentation. It has been found that DCs play a regulated role from taking up the antigen through processing and interacting with the T lymphocytes [105]. This interaction goes through a series of molecular events while deciding the fate of immune response at the inflammatory site [106]. DCs are present all through the lung milieu from nose to alveoli. The presence of these cells is such that they are found above and beneath the basement membrane of the respiratory epithelium putting them as first responders to incoming antigens [107]. Exogenously intruding antigens taken up either via endocytosis or phagocytosis are presented involving major histocompatibility complex (MHC) class II molecules to polarize $CD4^+$ T helper lymphocytes [106]. Studies using ovalbumin (OVA) sensitization mice model have demonstrated the role of DCs in promoting allergic inflammation and the clinical features of asthma by giving intraperitoneal injection of OVA in a Th2-inducing adjuvant, and repeated aerosol challenges resulted in lung eosinophilic infiltrates and enhanced secretion of mucus by airway epithelial cells and goblet cell hyperplasia [108]. Further, these changes were accompanied by airway obstruction and airway hyperresponsiveness after methacholine challenge, both of which are key features of asthma [109]. Significant escalation has been found in airway DCs after exposure to allergens in both murine and rat models of asthma [110–112]. In their functioning, the DCs are fitted out in such a fashion that they carry multiplicity of pattern recognition receptors (PPRs) for sensing the local environment, including Toll-like receptors (TLRs), NOD-like receptors, RIG-I-like receptors, and C-type lectin receptors [113, 114]. Activation of TLR4 has been found to help in initiating DC migration during recruitment of monocyte-derived $CD11b^+$ DCs to lungs in a house dust mite allergen mice model [110]. Reports have demonstrated that during ongoing inflammatory processes, DCs have a role in chemotaxis. Moreover, the DCs are able to produce CCL2, CCL3, CCL4, CCL17, TARC, CCL22, and CXCL8 [115]. Remarkably, production of CCR4 ligands (CCL17 and CCL22) by myeloid DCs suggests that these cells are capable of recruiting Th2 cells and/or $CD4^+$ $CD25^+$ regulatory cells at sites of inflammation during the late-phase asthmatic reaction [116].

2.5.2 Mast Cells

Mast cells originate from pluripotent hematopoietic stem cells, which circulate as $CD34^+$ precursors till they migrate into tissues for maturation and act as effector cells [117, 118]. Mast cells play a crucial role in the pathogenesis of asthma as their mediators have shown to cause bronchoconstriction. They are believed to be the central link between IgE and AHR [119, 120]. It has been found that patients with asthma had activated mucosal mast cells present at the airway surface and at airway smooth-muscle layer compared to healthy volunteers [121]. Further, it has been demonstrated that these cells infiltrate in the airway mucous glands [122]. Mast cells have shown to cause bronchoconstriction and airway remodeling by releasing histamine and tryptase [123]. Reports have revealed that the number of degranulated mast cells significantly increased in asthmatic patients [124, 125]. This degranulation of mast cells may be a part of allergens causing cross-linking of antigens by mast cell IgE antibodies on the FcεRI receptor as this cross-linking is well documented to initiate a signaling cascade and synthesis of pro-inflammatory molecules [126–129]. However, IgE-dependent mast-cell activation without cross-linking of FcεRI is still a controversially discussed mechanism of mast-cell activation. During mast-cell activation, single receptor-bound IgE molecules induce cytokine production even without cross-linking of FcεRI and regulate mast-cell homeostasis [117, 130, 131]. Mast cells can also be activated by numerous other stimuli, for example, Toll-like receptors and MAS-related G-protein-coupled receptor X2. Reports have revealed that isolated human bronchi with the ability to contract in response to allergens had a higher number of smooth-muscle-associated mast cells than unresponsive human bronchi isolates [124]. Furthermore, an increased number of mast cells were found in the distal airways of subjects with nonfatal and fatal asthma compared to nonasthmatic controls. Biopsies from patients with severe asthma have demonstrated that the number of MC_{TC} and the MC_{TC}/MC_T ratio in the small airways were higher compared to normal subjects. However, a positive correlation between MC_{TC} in the region of small airways/alveolar attachments and lung function was found, suggesting a protective role of this subtype of mast cells [132].

2.5.3 Eosinophils

Eosinophils are circulating granulocytes that develop and mature in the bone marrow from $CD34^+$ progenitor cells and are released to the peripheral blood as mature cells. These cells play a vital role as effector cells during the inflammatory cascade and are involved in pathogenesis of asthma [133]. Interleukin 5 (IL-5), IL-13, and CC chemokine receptor (CCR)3 have been found essentially in recruiting eosinophils to the lung during allergic inflammation and participate in the modulation of immune response, induction of airway hyperresponsiveness, and remodeling [134]. Differentiation, activation, and survival of eosinophils are largely regulated by IL-5. Reports have demonstrated that they regulate the allergen-dependent Th2 pulmonary immune responses mediated by dendritic cells and T lymphocytes, as well as suppress Th1 responses [135]. Furthermore, a direct relationship between eosinophil count and the frequency of asthma exacerbations has been found in patients with severe asthma [136, 137]. Eosinophils are associated with the development of AHR through the release of basic proteins and oxygen-derived free radicals. Their accumulation at the bronchial sites damages by degranulating and releasing toxic proteins such as eosinophil-derived neurotoxin, eosinophil cationic protein, eosinophil peroxidase, and major basic proteins [138]. It has been found that sputum eosinophilia is found among nearly half of all patients with asthma, and both blood and sputum eosinophilia are associated with more severe disease, worse control, and worse prognosis [139]. Furthermore, it has been found that blocking IL-5 via antibodies had a profound and prolonged reduction in circulating and sputum eosinophils [140]. Eosinophils have shown to release leukotrienes, growth factors, and metalloproteinases that are involved in airway remodeling. In addition, the leukotrienes liberated from mast cells and eosinophils are also potent bronchoconstrictors and prolong the migration of eosinophils to the airways [141–143].

2.5.4 Basophils

Basophils are derived from basophil/mast-cell precursor cells in the bone marrow, comprising less than 1% of the blood leukocytes, and share some characteristics with mast cells phenotypically and functionally, including basophilic granules in their cytoplasm and expression of the high-affinity IgE receptor FcεRI on their cell surfaces and working as effector cells in allergic airway inflammation [144–146]. They play critical roles in both IgE-dependent and IgE-independent allergic inflammation, through their migration to the site of inflammation and secretion of various mediators, including cytokines, chemokines, and proteases [147]. Studies using mouse model of allergic asthma have found that basophils highly expressed

OX40 ligand (OX40L) after activation, and interestingly, blockade of OX40–OX40L interaction suppressed basophil-primed Th2 cell differentiation in vitro and ameliorated ovalbumin (OVA)-induced allergic eosinophilic inflammation mediated by Th2 activation [147]. In addition, reports have found that R8 (a Vasicine analogue) was able to suppress the Th2 cytokine production and eosinophil recruitment to the airways and further decreased methacholine-induced AHR, Th2 cytokine release, infiltration of inflammatory cells into the airways, serum IgE levels in preventive OVA induced murine model of asthma [148]. Basophils play their role in early as well as late phases of asthma, and their number was found to be increased in lungs of the patients who died of asthma [149]. It has been found that depletion of basophils resulted in abolishing Th2 differentiation. Independent studies have found a role for basophils compared to DCs, for antigen presentation in driving Th2 differentiation. Basophils have been found to express both MHC-II and costimulatory molecules (CD80, CD86, or CD40) necessary for APC function and could process and present antigens to naïve T cells, leading to Th2 cell differentiation. Interestingly, depletion of basophils using anti-FcεRI antibody has abolished Th2 differentiation in vivo, whereas depletion of DCs using CD11c-DTR chimeric mice had no significant effects on Th2 differentiation in these models [150–152].

2.5.5 Neutrophils

Neutrophils are polymorphonuclear leukocytes that play an essential role in the immune system, acting as the first line of defense against bacterial and fungal infections. They are the first cells to be recruited to the site of the allergic reaction. In noneosinophilic phenotypes of asthma, neutrophils are the dominant subpopulation of inflammatory cells. Increased levels of neutrophils and interleukin 8 (IL-8) have been found in airways of asthmatic patients [153]. They have shown to release a variety of cytokines and chemokines which can influence airway remodeling. Neutrophils from asthmatic subjects revealed an increased expression of adhesion molecules, especially after allergen challenge [154]. Patients with symptomatic asthma have shown escalated levels of peripheral neutrophils that display signs of activated neutrophils. Both the numbers and activation levels of these neutrophils are lower in the absence of symptoms or after treatment [155]. Studies have shown increased neutrophil numbers in airway lavage from patients with severe asthma compared to normal individuals [156]. The activation of peripheral blood neutrophils results in their intravascular migration, adhesion to the endothelium, and migration to the site of inflammation. Nocturnal asthma is associated with higher levels of neutrophils, which correlate with the severity of the disease [104]. Neutrophils were found in sputum of some patients who died of sudden-onset asthma compared to eosinophils. Studies using sputum cell counts and lung function (FEV1 pre- and post-bronchodilator) in over 1100 patients with asthma have found that both high neutrophil numbers and high eosinophil numbers were associated with a low prebronchodilator FEV1, but only high neutrophil numbers were associated with a low postbronchodilator FEV1. Interestingly, they have further reported that there is a tenfold increase in neutrophil count which is associated with a 92-ml reduction in postbronchodilator FEV1, indicating that airway neutrophilia is a characteristic of more severe asthma [157].

2.5.6 Macrophages

Macrophages that are produced by the differentiation of blood monocytes are recruited to the airways during asthmatic conditions. They play dual role in allergic responses and inflammation in the airways. It has been found that they are recruited to the airways of allergic subjects following allergen challenge [158]. Macrophages are the most abundant leukocytes found in alveoli, distal airspaces, and conducting airways [159–161]. Alveolar macrophages are the first cells to encounter inhaled substances initiating a variety of mediators which may have a putative role in asthma. Numerous reports have suggested that there is a significant association between lung macrophages, airway remodeling, and eosinophilic inflammation in asthma [162, 163]. Alveolar macrophages have been found to regulate pro- and anti-inflammatory responses in the airways, suggesting their critical role in asthma. Recent studies have demonstrated that macrophages are not only associated with the maintenance of pulmonary homeostasis by performing anti-inflammatory functions but also play an integral part of the mechanisms perpetuating inflammation and tissue injury associated with asthma as well [164]. In the airway lumen and bronchial mucosa, macrophages are major cellular sources of critical pro-inflammatory cytokines, including TNF-α, IL-1β, IL-6, and IL-8 [165, 166]. Alveolar macrophages from asthmatic patients release more TNF-α, IL-1β, IL-6, and IL-8 than healthy controls, but exhibit a diminished inflammatory response to LPS stimulation. In contrast to healthy alveolar macrophages, IL-4 treatment fails to significantly inhibit LPS-induced pro-inflammatory cytokine release in asthmatic alveolar macrophages [167–169].

2.5.7 $CD4^+$ T Cells

Normally, the response toward allergens is tolerance, but in asthmatic patients, this response is with elevated Th2-type immune responses. Th2-type $CD4^+$ T cells have shown to secrete IL-4, IL-5, and IL-13, playing a crucial downstream role in pathogenesis of asthma [100]. Recent reports have demonstrated several features of $CD4^+$ T cells in the blood of atopic asthma patients like asthmatic patients who had a profound increase of $CCR7^+$ memory $CD4^+$ T cells, but not $CCR7^-$ memory $CD4^+$ T cells. There was an increase in $CCR4^+$ $CD4^+$ T cells in patients which is attributed to the increase of $CCR7^+$ memory $CD4^+$ T cells. Further patients had an increase of Tregs, as measured by quantifying CD25, Foxp3, IL-10, and CTLA-4 expression. However, asthma severity was inversely correlated only with the frequency of CTLA-4^+ $CD4^+$ T cells. Moreover, patients and control subjects have similar frequencies of $CD4^+$ T cells that express CCR5, CCR6, CXCR3, CXCR5,

CD11a, or α4 integrin. However, the frequency of $\alpha 4^{+}$ $CD4^{+}$ T cells in patients correlated with asthma severity [170]. Studies have shown that patients with allergic asthma and allergic subjects without asthma demonstrated escalated allergen-specific $CD4^{+}$ T-cell activation and IL-4 production from stimulated peripheral blood mononuclear cells (PBMCs) compared with healthy control subjects [171, 172]. However, patients with allergic asthma produced more IL-5 from stimulated PBMCs or bronchoalveolar lavage compared to either allergic subjects without asthma or healthy control subjects [173]. Further, the studies have revealed that IL-5 production by $CD4^{+}$ T cells could be improved by alveolar macrophages from subjects with allergic asthma but not allergic subjects without asthma [174, 175]. Studies in human subjects have revealed that levels of Th2 cytokines, including IL-4, IL-5, and IL-13, are elevated in the airways of subjects with asthma at baseline and after allergen challenge [176]. Increased expression of Th2 transcription factors STAT6 (signal transducer and activator of transcription-6) and GATA3 (GATA-binding protein-3) has been detected in bronchial biopsies of asthmatic patients [177, 178].

2.5.8 $CD8^{+}$ Tc2 Cells

In contrast to $CD4^{+}$ T cells, the role of $CD8^{+}$ T cells is suggested to balance the responses of $CD4^{+}$ T cells through the secretion of interferon (IFN)-γ [179]. In humans, Tc2 cells have revealed predominant presence in fatal asthma, while in stable states, severe eosinophilic asthma is associated with greater numbers of Tc2 than Th2 cells in blood, bronchoalveolar lavage fluid, and bronchial biopsies [180]. $CD8^{+}$ T cells have been found to play a crucial role in asthma pathogenesis largely due to their insensitivity toward corticosteroids compared to $CD4^{+}$ T cells and because they have the capacity to undergo transcriptional reprogramming from IFN-γ-secreting cells (Tc1) to type 2 cytokine secreting cells (Tc2), especially producing IL-13 and IL-5 [181]. Depletion of $CD8^{+}$ T cells attenuated AHR and airway inflammation in mice exposed to allergen exclusively via the airways in the absence of systemic sensitization [182]. Significant activation of circulating $CD8^{+}$ T cells in peripheral blood has been found in severe asthma and linked with downregulation of specific microRNAs (miR-146a/b and miR-28-5p) and differential expression of multiple intronic long noncoding RNAs, which might regulate $CD8^{+}$ T-cell activities [183]. Tc2 cells strongly express CRTH2, the receptor for prostaglandin D2, the cysteinyl leukotriene receptor 1, and the leukotriene B4 receptor. When activated, these elicit Tc2 cell chemotaxis and production of chemokines and type 2 and other cytokines, resulting directly or indirectly in eosinophil recruitment and survival [184].

2.6 Transcriptional Regulation of Asthma

Over recent past, Th1/Th2 paradigm has offered significant insights for investigating the pathogenesis of asthma, and there is an accord that the central underlying pathology of the disease is chronic airway inflammation involving inflammatory cells, such as Th2 lymphocytes and eosinophils [185]. In most of the allergic conditions and asthmatic patients, activated Th2 cells secrete numerous cytokines and inflammatory mediators that provoke the inflammatory response. Among these, the cytokines IL-4, IL-5, and IL-13 are responsible for many of the features of allergic inflammation [186, 187]. Studies have revealed that the transcription factors that are involved in asthmatic inflammation and control the expression and function of these cytokines include signal transducer and activator of transcription 6, cyclic AMP response element-binding protein (CREB), GATA3, nuclear factor of activated T cells, and nuclear factor kB [188, 189]. Transcription factors have diverse functions, and their interaction may be important in amplifying and inhibiting the inflammatory process, making them a therapeutic target against allergic conditions and asthma.

2.6.1 NF-κB

NF-κB is a ubiquitous transcription factor having a vital role in inflammatory and immune responses. There is a precedent of literature indicating that NF-κB plays a crucial role in orchestrating the inflammatory response and acts as an amplifying and perpetuating mechanism [190]. Escalating expression levels of NF-κB signaling has been revealed in bronchial biopsies from asthmatic patients and in animal models of asthma [191–194]. Using mouse models, it has been found that NF-κB knockout mice were unable to mount Th2 responses because the T cells were not able to induce GATA3 expression, even under TH2-inducing conditions, and further, the mice that were deficient in NF-κB p50 or p65 had no eosinophilia and airway inflammation [195–197]. In addition, antisense phosphorothioate oligonucleotides directed at NF-κB p65 in a murine model of asthma have shown to inhibit allergic inflammation, including decrease in airway hyperresponsiveness and reduced Th2 cytokine production [198]. It has been found that NF-κB may be activated in vitro by diverse signals that exacerbate asthmatic inflammation like allergen exposure, rhinovirus infection, pro-inflammatory cytokines, and oxidants [199]. A recent study has shown that the nuclear translocation of phosphorylated P65, the inhibition of IκB kinase (IKK) within the NF-κB signaling pathway, and activation of the MAPK signaling pathway can control the production of IgE and IL-4 and inhibit inflammatory mediators in asthma [200].

2.6.2 STAT6

The signal transducer and activator of transcription (STAT) play a vital role during the selective response to cytokines [201]. STAT proteins undergo phosphorylation by the Janus family of kinases once they are stimulated by the cytokines. IL-4 arrangement with its receptor leads to phosphorylation of STAT6 by Jak1 and Jak3 and results in the activation of IL-4-regulated genes, such as IL-4R, IgE, FcR, and MHC class II molecules [201]. IL-4 has shown to play a crucial role in driving Th2 cell differentiation, and therefore, STAT6 is a critical transcription factor in this process. In humans, there is an alternate pathway for STAT6 via IL-13 [202]. It has been found that although IL-4$^{-/-}$ mice have residual Th2 responses, STAT6$^{-/-}$ mice had more or less complete abolition of Th2 responses. In murine models of allergic inflammation, STAT6$^{-/-}$ mice revealed noticeable attenuation of pulmonary eosinophilia, mucus production, AHR, and serum IgE levels [203]. Moreover, other similar studies have shown that STAT6 knockout mice do not have Th2 cells, and there is no class switching to IgE, thus demonstrating the essential role of STAT6 [204–206]. Studies using murine models of contact hypersensitivity and atopic dermatitis have shown that STAT6 deficiency results in abrogation of IL-4- and IL-13-dependent inflammation, with decreased eosinophilia, edema, and IgE responses in both models [207, 208]. In vitro studies using antisense phosphorothioate oligodeoxynucleotides targeting STAT6 have been found promising in suppressing STAT6 signaling in airway smooth-muscle and epithelial cell lines [209, 210]. Selective STAT6 blockers are also under preclinical trials, and some of them have already shown promising effects in animal models of asthma [211, 212]. Assuming the role of STAT6 in all aspects of IL-4 and IL-13 signaling, local blockade of STAT6 function remains a very promising approach for the treatment of allergic diseases.

2.6.3 GATA3

GATA-3 belongs to the GATA family of transcription factors, which bind to the WGATAR (W = A/T; R = A/G) DNA sequence through a highly conserved C4 zinc-finger domain. It was first reported as a transcription factor that interacted with the TCR-α gene enhancer [213]. In addition to its essential role in T-cell development, GATA-3 has also been identified as a Th2 differentiation factor. Significant increase in GATA-3 expression has been revealed in asthmatic airways compared to control subjects, and this escalated expression has been correlated significantly with IL-5 expression and AHR [177]. GATA3 is thought to function via chromatin remodeling of the Th2 cytokine locus, binding at multiple sites and therefore allowing Th2 cells to express IL-4, IL-5, and IL-13 [214, 215]. It has been demonstrated that Th2 cells play an important role in the pathogenesis of the asthma when primarily mediated through the cytokine IL-13, and inhibiting GATA3 activity or blocking its expression may attenuate the interleukin-13-mediated asthma phenotypes [216]. Overexpression of GATA3 in T cells has shown to induce Th2 cytokine expression in both naive cells and dedicated Th1 cells in both mice and human subjects [217, 218]. Inhibition of GATA-3 activity has demonstrated to cause a severe dampening of Th2 effects, both locally (eosinophil influx and mucus production) and systemically (IgE production) in lungs [219]. Studies using murine models have shown that transgenic mice overexpressing GATA3 in T cells show enhanced airway hyperresponsiveness, smooth-muscle hyperplasia, and increased subepithelial fibrosis [220, 221]. Lentiviral particles expressing GATA3 siRNA were delivered intratracheally, and it was found to alleviate airway eosinophilia, Th2 cytokine production, and airway hyperresponsiveness. Similarly, siRNA-targeting GATA3 in human T cells has also been shown to downregulate Th2 cytokine production, signifying that this may be a possible therapeutic approach [222]. R8 (a Vasicine analogue) has shown significant decrease in Th2 cytokine secretion and eosinophilia and further decreased the phosphorylation levels of STAT6 and expression of GATA3 in murine model of asthma [223].

2.6.4 NFAT

Nuclear factor of activated T cells (NFAT) is a family of five members (NFAT1-5), transcription factors where four of these are regulated by calcium signaling (NFAT1-4) [224, 225]. NFAT-induced inflammation is a well-recognized player in asthma pathogenesis. It has been shown to play an important role in transcription of the Th2 cytokine genes during T-cell activation in coordination with other transcription factors, such as activator protein 1 (AP-1), GATA3, and c-Maf [226]. Mice models that were deficient of NFAT1 and NFAT2 had revealed profound defects in T-cell cytokine production, including IL-4 and IL-5 production [227]. Reports have demonstrated that the activation of Ca^{2+}/NFAT signaling events significantly contributed to the release of thymic stromal lymphopoietin (TSLP) from airway epithelial cells [228]. Moreover, the activation of the Ca^{2+} release-activated Ca^{2+} (CRAC) channel/NFAT pathway in airway epithelial cells had led to the production of multiple inflammatory mediators, including TSLP, interleukin (IL)-6, and prostaglandin E2 [229]. In addition, the exposure of airway epithelial cells to house dust mite resulted in the activation of protease-activated receptor type 2 (PAR2), opening of CRAC channels, and upregulation of downstream NFAT signaling pathways [230]. The immunosuppressive drugs cyclosporin A (CsA), FK506 (tacrolimus), and pimecrolimus have shown to block calcineurin-dependent dephosphorylation of NFAT through their cellular receptors cyclophilin and FK506-binding protein, but it had a little success, so more specific NFAT antagonists are needed to target this signaling pathway.

2.7 Current Treatment for Asthma, Drawbacks, and Future Directions

Asthma management is largely guided by the Global Initiative for Asthma (GINA) strategy and is based on a mainstay of inhaled corticosteroid (ICS) therapy along with additional therapeutic candidates to achieve disease control. Although the mechanistic studies have greatly improved our understanding of molecular and cellular components involved in asthma and our ability to treat severe patients, however, a major proportion of patients with symptomatic asthma remain uncontrolled. The long-term goals of asthma management are symptom control, minimizing the risk of exacerbations in future, and reduction of airflow limitation while concurrently minimizing treatment side effects [231]. A large prospective trial verified that adherence to an existing schedule of high-dose inhaled corticosteroid (ICS) with long-acting beta-adrenergic agonist has resulted in well-controlled asthma in approximately 60% of patients with severe uncontrolled asthma [232].

2.7.1 New Treatment Recommendations

The 2019 GINA strategy report symbolized the most important change in asthma management in 30 years. For safety reasons, GINA no longer recommends treatment with short-acting beta 2-agonists (SABA) alone. There is strong evidence that SABA-only treatment, although providing short-term relief of asthma symptoms, does not protect patients from severe exacerbations, and that regular or frequent use of SABAs increases the risk of exacerbations. GINA now recommends that all adults and adolescents with asthma should receive either symptom-driven (in mild asthma) or daily low-dose ICS-containing controller treatment, to reduce their risk of serious exacerbations [233].

2.7.2 Long-Term Asthma Control

Daily use of medications for long-term control (LTC) of symptoms is the keystone of care in controlling asthma symptoms and preventing recurrent exacerbations of asthma for most of the patients [234]. A recent study has shown that by using 5 years of Behavioral Risk Factor Surveillance System (BRFSS) Child and Adult Asthma Call-back Survey (ACBS) data, among the current patients with asthma, 46.0% of children and 41.5% of adults were taking LTC medications and 38.4% of children and 50.0% of adults had uncontrolled asthma. Among children who had uncontrolled asthma (38.4%), 24.1% were taking LTC medications and 14.3% were not taking LTC medications. Among adults who had uncontrolled asthma (50.0%), 26.7% were taking LTC medications and 23.3% were not taking LTC medications [235].

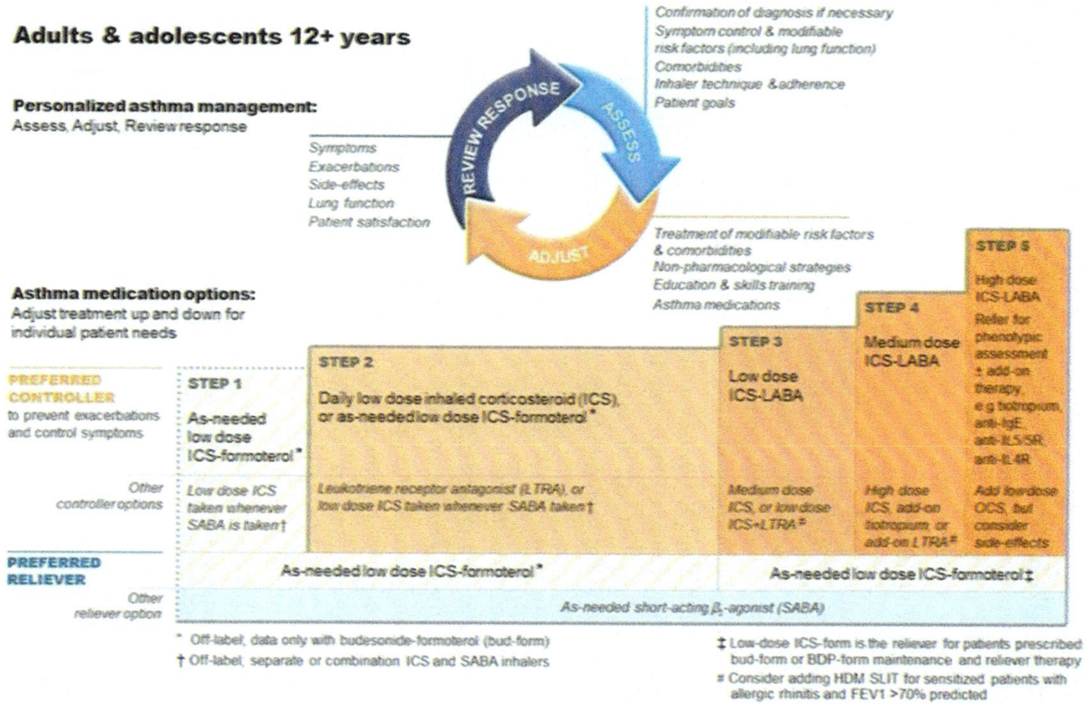

The GINA asthma treatment strategy. (GINA 2019 report (www.ginasthma.org))

2.7.2.1 Inhaled Corticosteroids

Corticosteroids are anti-inflammatory agents that suppress Th2-mediated inflammation by modulating the expression of those cytokines, adhesion molecules, and chemokines that are under the transcriptional regulation of nuclear factor-κB (NFκB) and activator protein-1 (AP-1). They are one of the most widely used classes of medications to treat asthma, with broad anti-inflammatory and immunosuppressive effects. Inhaled corticosteroids (ICSs) are the most effective long-term control medication across all ages and are very effective in decreasing AHR with amelioration in asthma symptoms, pulmonary function, and reduction in morbidity. Moreover, it presents significantly less side effects and is generally safe for long-term use because of limited systemic absorption compared to oral corticosteroid therapy [236]. The anti-inflammatory drugs that are currently in use as ICSs include fluticasone (Flonase, Flovent HFA), budesonide (Pulmicort Flexhaler, Rhinocort), flunisolide (Aerospan HFA), ciclesonide (Alvesco, Omnaris, Zetonna), beclomethasone (Qnasl, Qvar), mometasone (Asmanex), and fluticasone furoate (Arnuity Ellipta) [237]. Inhaled corticosteroids can cause hoarseness, throat irritation, and a cough. Thrush (candidiasis), a yeast infection of the mouth and tongue, is another risk, especially in older individuals. However, it could be minimized by rinsing the mouth after inhalation, keeping the inhaler clean, and using a spacer device to reduce the amount of medicine that settles in mouth. In addition, studies have demonstrated a modest risk of cataracts, due to high dosage and long duration of use, consistent with the systemic absorption of ICS [238].

2.7.2.2 Leukotriene Modifiers

Leukotriene receptor antagonists (LTRAs) are believed to decrease edema, inflammation, and bronchoconstriction by inhibiting the binding of cysteinyl leukotrienes to their corresponding receptors on both pro-inflammatory cells and smooth muscle [239, 240]. According to National Asthma Education and Prevention Program (NAEPP) guidelines, leukotriene receptor modifiers (LTMs) include adjunctive or alternative therapy in mild-to-severe persistent asthma. LTMs seem to be lesser monotherapy for controlling persistent asthma compared to ICSs, but they may play a vital role while treating the patients with aspirin-exacerbated respiratory disease as they are well tolerated with a favorable safety profile [241, 242]. LTRAs are recommended as alternative controller medications for adults with mild persistent asthma. LTRAs may reduce the dose of inhaled corticosteroids required by patients with moderate-to-severe asthma and may improve asthma control in individuals whose asthma is not controlled with a low dose or high dose of inhaled corticosteroids when it is used as add-on therapy. The use of LTRAs as a steroid-sparing treatment is encouraged in clinical practice [243]. The oral medications in this group that are currently in use include montelukast (Singulair), zafirlukast (Accolate), and zileuton (Zyflo). They help in relieving asthma symptoms for up to 24 h. In rare cases, these medications have been linked to psychological reactions, such as agitation, aggression, hallucinations, depression, and suicidal thinking.

2.7.2.3 Short-Acting Beta-2 Agonists

β2-adrenoceptor agonists are a class of drugs, commonly known as bronchodilators, that act by causing smooth-muscle relaxation via β2-adrenergic receptors. Currently, short-acting β2-adrenoceptor agonists are the most effective bronchodilators available for quick and transient relief. They are the first-line treatment for mild intermittent asthma, either salbutamol or terbutaline, taken by inhalation [244, 245]. Short-acting beta-2 agonists work on the beta-2 adrenergic receptors in the smooth muscle of bronchial tissue, producing bronchodilaton and relieving the symptoms of chest tightness and breathlessness [246]. Some of the adverse events due to these drugs include tachycardia and palpitations possibly due to beta stimulation and reflex cardiac stimulation.

2.7.2.4 Long-Acting Muscarinic Antagonists (Tiotropium Bromide)

Asthma management in children and teenagers is a complex balancing act between diagnosis, treatment, patient education, and adherence. Tiotropium has emerged as a promising new drug candidate as add-on therapy for the management of asthma in patients with partially controlled symptoms of all ages. Data from numerous clinical trials in patients aged 1–75 years with asthma demonstrated that the efficacy of tiotropium is consistent in both adults and children, irrespective of disease severity and phenotype [247]. The recent success of phase III pediatric trials led to the approval of tiotropium for the treatment of asthma in patients aged ≥6 years in the European Union and the United States [248]. Preclinical studies have demonstrated that tiotropium is effective in asthma, irrespective of baseline characteristics and phenotypes [249], and able to prevent airway remodeling and reduce airway inflammation [250–252]. Based on the evidences from the clinical trials in about 6000 patients across the age groups, tiotropium was found efficacious add-on therapy, with safety and tolerability comparable with placebo in the individual studies. Tiotropium is specified for once-daily use in the European Union (two inhalations of 2.5 μg) and the United States (two inhalations of 1.25 μg) as maintenance treatment in patients with severe asthma aged ≥6 years [253, 254].

2.7.2.5 Short-Acting Muscarinic Antagonists

Ipratropium bromide is a short-acting muscarinic antagonist that blocks M1, M2, and M3 muscarinic receptors nonselectively in the airways and exerts a bronchodilator effect in patients with asthma [255, 256]. Studies have reported that ipratropium resulted in significant improvements in bronchodilation after 4 weeks of treatment with bromide/albuterol combination therapy compared with albuterol alone, and it has been recommended as an alternative reliever agent for adult patients who are unable to tolerate treatment with SABAs [257, 258]. Studies have demonstrated that triple therapy with ipratropium, albuterol, and an OCS revealed considerable improvements in lung function compared with standard therapy in children with severe asthma exacerbation [256]. Moreover, ipratropium has been shown to be more effective in adults with nonatopic asthma and a longer duration of the disease [259]. However, some reports have demonstrated that ipratropium bromide is associated with an increased risk of adverse cardiovascular effects [260, 261].

2.7.2.6 IgE-Binding Antibodies

Omalizumab was developed in the 1990s and approved by FDA in 2003 for patients with severe persistent asthma >12 years of age. It is a biologically engineered, humanized recombinant monoclonal anti-IgE antibody inhibiting IgE functions by blocking free serum IgE and inhibiting their binding to cellular receptors like FcεRI. Recent studies have shown that specific binding of IgE by omalizumab reduces both the early allergic response and the late allergic response and symptoms of IgE-mediated allergy. The long-term clinical efficacy of omalizumab has been demonstrated along with improvements in quality of life. As add-on therapy in severe asthma, omalizumab reduces the requirement for inhaled corticosteroids and improves disease control. Clinical studies have shown that the patients who benefit most from omalizumab therapy are those at high risk of exacerbations, those with poorly controlled and/or severe asthma, and those with IgE-mediated comorbidities [262]. Anti-IgE antibodies have shown to decrease serum IgE levels in a dose-dependent manner and allergen-induced bronchoconstriction during both the early- and late-phase responses to inhaled allergen in atopic asthma patients [263–265]. Studies have demonstrated that considerable percentage of severe asthmatics revealed reduction in original bronchial RBM thickness and eosinophil infiltration after 1-year treatment with anti-IgE [266], and further, more a clinical study has shown that 16 weeks of treatment with omalizumab reduced airway wall thickness in asthmatic patients [267]. Reports have shown that IgE receptors on basophils and mast cells are downregulated with long-term use of omalizumab [268]. Omalizumab injections are generally well tolerated, but local skin reactions are common. Additionally, there is a 0.09% risk of anaphylaxis [269].

2.7.2.7 Mast-Cell Stabilizers (Cromolyn)

Cromolyn is the most widely used mast-cell stabilizer and a promising choice for asthma treatment due to its potent anti-inflammatory effects. According to the NAEPP guidelines, cromolyn is indicated as an alternative to ICS in mild persistent asthma [270]. It has shown to inhibit the immunoglobulin E (IgE)-mediated release of inflammatory mediators by mast cells in a dose-dependent fashion [271, 272]. Cromolyn is generally well tolerated and has few side effects. However, it requires four times daily administration, which has largely limited its clinical use.

2.8 Conclusion

Asthma is a chronic disease of airways, characterized by inflammation and accompanied with airway hyperresponsiveness, resulting in incidents of breathlessness, chest tightness, wheezing, and cough. It confers a substantial burden on individual's quality of life, as well as on global health and socioeconomics. Despite inordinate steps toward the management and treatment of this disease, there are still a good number of patients who remain difficult to control. Although the genetic factors, environmental influences, and specific trigger factors are implicated in the development of the disease, still we are in need to understand the cause, biology, and pathophysiology of the disease to come up with new treatment regimens which may decrease the burden of the patients and improve their quality of life. Great progress has been made recently in the development of targeted, phenotype-specific asthma therapies; however, all five of the biologic therapies approved for asthma address T2 inflammation, which has raised an urgent need to develop new therapeutic strategies for patients with non-T2 inflammation, who are least likely to be responsive to ICS therapeutic approach.

References

1. Akinbami LJ, Moorman JE, Liu X et al (2012) NCHS Data Brief (94):1–8
2. Akinbami LJ, Moorman JE, Liu X (2011) National health statistics reports. National Center for Health Statistics, Hyattsville, MD, pp 2005–2009
3. National Heart, Lung, and Blood Institute (NHLBI) of the National Institutes of Health (2007) National Asthma Education and Prevention Program Expert Panel Report 3 (EPR-3): Guidelines for the diagnosis and management of asthma—Summary report 2007. National Institutes of Health (NIH) Publication (08-5846)
4. Bateman ED et al (2008) Global strategy for asthma management and prevention: GINA executive summary. Eur Respir J 31(1):143–178
5. Martinez FD et al (1995) Asthma and wheezing in the first six years of life. N Engl J Med 332 (3):133–138
6. Lowe LA et al (2005) Wheeze phenotypes and lung function in preschool children. Am J Respir Crit Care Med 171(3):231–237
7. Young S et al (2000) The association between early life lung function and wheezing during the first 2 yrs of life. Eur Respir J 15(1):151–157
8. Bauer BA et al (1997) Incidence and outcomes of asthma in the elderly: a population-based study in Rochester, Minnesota. Chest 111(2):303–310
9. Butland BK, Strachan DP (2007) Asthma onset and relapse in adult life: the British 1958 birth cohort study. Ann Allergy Asthma Immunol 98(4):337–343
10. Wenzel SE (2006) Asthma: defining of the persistent adult phenotypes. Lancet 368 (9537):804–813
11. Gilliland FD et al (2006) Regular smoking and asthma incidence in adolescents. Am J Respir Crit Care Med 174(10):1094–1100
12. Tetrault JM et al (2007) Effects of marijuana smoking on pulmonary function and respiratory complications: a systematic review. Arch Intern Med 167(3):221–228
13. Taylor DR et al (2002) A longitudinal study of the effects of tobacco and cannabis exposure on lung function in young adults. Addiction 97(8):1055–1061
14. McCreanor J et al (2007) Respiratory effects of exposure to diesel traffic in persons with asthma. N Engl J Med 357(23):2348–2358
15. Bakerly ND et al (2008) Fifteen-year trends in occupational asthma: data from the Shield surveillance scheme. Occup Med 58(3):169–174
16. Willemsen G et al (2008) Heritability of self-reported asthma and allergy: a study in adult Dutch twins, siblings and parents. Twin Res Hum Genet 11(2):132–142
17. Holberg CJ et al (1996) Segregation analysis of physician-diagnosed asthma in Hispanic and non-Hispanic white families. A recessive component? Am J Respir Crit Care Med 154 (1):144–150
18. Lawrence S et al (1994) Genetic analysis of atopy and asthma as quantitative traits and ordered polychotomies. Ann Hum Genet 58(4):359–368
19. Stein RT et al (1999) Influence of parental smoking on respiratory symptoms during the first decade of life: the Tucson Children's Respiratory Study. Am J Epidemiol 149(11):1030–1037

20. Lewis S et al (1995) Prospective study of risk factors for early and persistent wheezing in childhood. Eur Respir J 8(3):349–356
21. Lau S et al (2002) The development of childhood asthma: lessons from the German Multicentre Allergy Study (MAS). Paediatr Respir Rev 3(3):265–272
22. Tariq S et al (2000) Influence of smoking on asthmatic symptoms and allergen sensitisation in early childhood. Postgrad Med J 76(901):694–699
23. Willers S et al (2007) Maternal food consumption during pregnancy and asthma, respiratory and atopic symptoms in 5-year-old children. Thorax 62(9):773–779
24. Romieu I et al (2007) Maternal fish intake during pregnancy and atopy and asthma in infancy. Clin Exp Allergy 37(4):518–525
25. Mihrshahi S et al (2007) The association between infant feeding practices and subsequent atopy among children with a family history of asthma. Clin Exp Allergy 37(5):671–679
26. Nafstad P, Magnus P, Jaakkola JJ (2000) Risk of childhood asthma and allergic rhinitis in relation to pregnancy complications. J Allergy Clin Immunol 106(5):867–873
27. Annesi-Maesano I, Moreau D, Strachan D (2001) In utero and perinatal complications preceding asthma. Allergy 56(6):491–497
28. Lewis S et al (1996) Study of the aetiology of wheezing illness at age 16 in two national British birth cohorts. Thorax 51(7):670–676
29. Stick SM et al (1996) Effects of maternal smoking during pregnancy and a family history of asthma on respiratory function in newborn infants. Lancet 348(9034):1060–1064
30. Asher MI, Ellwood P (2014) The global asthma report 2014. Global Asthma Network, New Zealand
31. Lugogo NL, Kraft M (2006) Epidemiology of asthma. Clin Chest Med 27(1):1–15
32. Bousquet J, Humbert M (2015) GINA 2015: the latest iteration of a magnificent journey. Eur Respir J 46:579–582
33. Ferkol T, Schraufnagel D (2014) The global burden of respiratory disease. Ann Am Thorac Soc 11(3):404–406
34. Wang D et al (2013) Cross-sectional epidemiological survey of asthma in Jinan, China. Respirology 18(2):313–322
35. Burney P, Jarvis D, Perez-Padilla R (2015) The global burden of chronic respiratory disease in adults. Int J Tuberc Lung Dis 19(1):10–20
36. Sears MR (2014) Trends in the prevalence of asthma. Chest 145(2):219–225
37. Baïz N, Annesi-Maesano I (2012) Is the asthma epidemic still ascending? Clin Chest Med 33 (3):419–429
38. Aaron SD et al (2008) Overdiagnosis of asthma in obese and nonobese adults. CMAJ 179 (11):1121–1131
39. Bauer UE et al (2014) Prevention of chronic disease in the 21st century: elimination of the leading preventable causes of premature death and disability in the USA. Lancet 384 (9937):45–52
40. Dharmage SC, Perret J, Custovic A (2019) Epidemiology of asthma in children and adults. Front Pediatr 7:246
41. Nurmagambetov T, Kuwahara R, Garbe P (2018) The economic burden of asthma in the United States, 2008–2013. Ann Am Thorac Soc 15(3):348–356
42. Schiller JS, Lucas JW, Peregoy JA (2012) Summary health statistics for US adults: national health interview survey, 2011. Vital Health Stat (252):1–207
43. Netuveli G et al (2005) Ethnic variations in UK asthma frequency, morbidity, and health-service use: a systematic review and meta-analysis. Lancet 365(9456):312–317
44. Sheikh A et al (2016) Ethnic variations in asthma hospital admission, readmission and death: a retrospective, national cohort study of 4.62 million people in Scotland. BMC Med 14(1):3
45. Wang H-Y et al (2008) Prevalence of asthma among Chinese adolescents living in Canada and in China. CMAJ 179(11):1133–1142
46. To T et al (2012) Global asthma prevalence in adults: findings from the cross-sectional world health survey. BMC Public Health 12(1):204

47. Wong GW, Leung TF, Ko FW (2013) Changing prevalence of allergic diseases in the Asia-pacific region. Allergy, Asthma Immunol Res 5(5):251–257
48. Global Asthma Network Group (2014) The global asthma report 2014. Global Asthma Network Group, Auckland, New Zealand, p 769
49. Schluger NW, Koppaka R (2014) Lung disease in a global context. A call for public health action. Ann Am Thorac Soc 11(3):407–416
50. Asher I, Pearce N (2014) Global burden of asthma among children. Int J Tuberc Lung Dis 18 (11):1269–1278
51. Adeloye D et al (2013) An estimate of asthma prevalence in Africa: a systematic analysis. Croat Med J 54(6):519–531
52. Holgate ST (2012) Innate and adaptive immune responses in asthma. Nat Med 18(5):673
53. Erle DJ, Sheppard D (2014) The cell biology of asthma. J Cell Biol 205(5):621–631
54. Kudo M, Ishigatsubo Y, Aoki I (2013) Pathology of asthma. Front Microbiol 4:263
55. van der Meer A-N et al (2016) A 1-day visit in a severe asthma centre: effect on asthma control, quality of life and healthcare use. Eur Respir J 48(3):726–733
56. Hogg JC (1997) The pathology of asthma. APMIS 105(7–12):735–745
57. Hamid Q et al (1997) Inflammation of small airways in asthma. J Allergy Clin Immunol 100 (1):44–51
58. Martin RJ (1998) Small airway and alveolar tissue changes in nocturnal asthma. Am J Respir Crit Care Med 157(5):S188–S190
59. Demedts IK et al (2005) Matrix metalloproteinases in asthma and COPD. Curr Opin Pharmacol 5(3):257–263
60. Moreno RH, Hogg JC, Paré PD (1986) Mechanics of airway narrowing. Am Rev Respir Dis 133(6):1171–1180
61. James AL, Paré PD, Hogg JC (1989) The mechanics of airway narrowing in asthma. Am Rev Respir Dis 139(1):242–246
62. Pare P et al (1997) The functional consequences of airway remodeling in asthma. Monaldi Arch Chest Dis 52(6):589–596
63. Ebina M et al (1993) Cellular hypertrophy and hyperplasia of airway smooth muscle underlying bronchial asthma. Am Rev Respir Dis 148:720–726
64. James AL et al (2012) Airway smooth muscle hypertrophy and hyperplasia in asthma. Am J Respir Crit Care Med 185(10):1058–1064
65. Oliver MN et al (2007) Airway hyperresponsiveness, remodeling, and smooth muscle mass: right answer, wrong reason? Am J Respir Cell Mol Biol 37(3):264–272
66. Elliot JG et al (2015) Distribution of airway smooth muscle remodelling in asthma: relation to airway inflammation. Respirology 20(1):66–72
67. Carroll N et al (1996) Airway structure and inflammatory cells in fatal attacks of asthma. Eur Respir J 9(4):709–715
68. Faul J et al (1997) Lung immunopathology in cases of sudden asthma death. Eur Respir J 10 (2):301–307
69. Kraft M et al (1999) Lymphocyte and eosinophil influx into alveolar tissue in nocturnal asthma. Am J Respir Crit Care Med 159(1):228–234
70. Mauad T et al (2004) Abnormal alveolar attachments with decreased elastic fiber content in distal lung in fatal asthma. Am J Respir Crit Care Med 170(8):857–862
71. Gelb AF et al (2002) Unsuspected loss of lung elastic recoil in chronic persistent asthma. Chest 121(3):715–721
72. Holgate S et al (1999) The bronchial epithelium as a key regulator of airway inflammation and remodelling in asthma. Clin Exp Allergy 29:90–95
73. Reddel CJ, Weiss AS, Burgess JK (2012) Elastin in asthma. Pulm Pharmacol Ther 25 (2):144–153
74. Holtzman MJ et al (2014) The role of airway epithelial cells and innate immune cells in chronic respiratory disease. Nat Rev Immunol 14(10):686–698

75. Puddicombe S et al (2000) Involvement of the epidermal growth factor receptor in epithelial repair in asthma. FASEB J 14(10):1362–1374
76. Lambrecht BN, Hammad H (2012) The airway epithelium in asthma. Nat Med 18(5):684
77. Knight DA et al (2001) Protease-activated receptors in human airways: upregulation of PAR-2 in respiratory epithelium from patients with asthma. J Allergy Clin Immunol 108(5):797–803
78. Barnes PJ et al (2009) Asthma and COPD: basic mechanisms and clinical management. Elsevier, Amsterdam
79. Holgate ST et al (2000) Epithelial-mesenchymal interactions in the pathogenesis of asthma. J Allergy Clin Immunol 105(2):193–204
80. Doeing DC, Solway J (2013) Airway smooth muscle in the pathophysiology and treatment of asthma. J Appl Physiol 114(7):834–843
81. James AL et al (2009) Airway smooth muscle thickness in asthma is related to severity but not duration of asthma. Eur Respir J 34(5):1040–1045
82. Benayoun L et al (2003) Airway structural alterations selectively associated with severe asthma. Am J Respir Crit Care Med 167(10):1360–1368
83. Pepe C et al (2005) Differences in airway remodeling between subjects with severe and moderate asthma. J Allergy Clin Immunol 116(3):544–549
84. Berair R, Hollins F, Brightling C (2013) Airway smooth muscle hypercontractility in asthma. J Allergy 2013:185971
85. Damera G, Tliba O, Panettieri RA Jr (2009) Airway smooth muscle as an immunomodulatory cell. Pulm Pharmacol Ther 22(5):353–359
86. Lazaar AL, Panettieri RA Jr (2005) Airway smooth muscle: a modulator of airway remodeling in asthma. J Allergy Clin Immunol 116(3):488–495
87. Fernandes DJ et al (2003) Invited Review: Do inflammatory mediators influence the contribution of airway smooth muscle contraction to airway hyperresponsiveness in asthma? J Appl Physiol 95(2):844–853
88. Brightling CE et al (2002) Mast-cell infiltration of airway smooth muscle in asthma. N Engl J Med 346(22):1699–1705
89. Rogers DF, Barnes PJ (2006) Treatment of airway mucus hypersecretion. Ann Med 38 (2):116–125
90. Martínez-Rivera C et al (2018) Mucus hypersecretion in asthma is associated with rhinosinusitis, polyps and exacerbations. Respir Med 135:22–28
91. Williams OW et al (2006) Airway mucus: from production to secretion. Am J Respir Cell Mol Biol 34(5):527–536
92. Kuyper LM et al (2003) Characterization of airway plugging in fatal asthma. Am J Med 115 (1):6–11
93. Wagers SS et al (2007) Intrinsic and antigen-induced airway hyperresponsiveness are the result of diverse physiological mechanisms. J Appl Physiol 102(1):221–230
94. Wan H et al (2004) Foxa2 regulates alveolarization and goblet cell hyperplasia. Development 131(4):953–964
95. Ordoñez CL et al (2001) Mild and moderate asthma is associated with airway goblet cell hyperplasia and abnormalities in mucin gene expression. Am J Respir Crit Care Med 163 (2):517–523
96. Dillard P, Wetsel RA, Drouin SM (2007) Complement C3a regulates Muc5ac expression by airway Clara cells independently of Th2 responses. Am J Respir Crit Care Med 175 (12):1250–1258
97. Song JS et al (2007) Nitric oxide induces MUC5AC mucin in respiratory epithelial cells through PKC and ERK dependent pathways. Respir Res 8(1):28
98. Lora JM et al (2005) Tumor necrosis factor-α triggers mucus production in airway epithelium through an IκB kinase β-dependent mechanism. J Biol Chem 280(43):36510–36517
99. Perrais M et al (2002) Induction of MUC2 and MUC5AC mucins by factors of the epidermal growth factor (EGF) family is mediated by EGF receptor/Ras/Raf/extracellular signal-regulated kinase cascade and Sp1. J Biol Chem 277(35):32258–32267

100. Barrett NA, Austen KF (2009) Innate cells and T helper 2 cell immunity in airway inflammation. Immunity 31(3):425–437
101. Melis M et al (2002) Fluticasone induces apoptosis in peripheral T-lymphocytes: a comparison between asthmatic and normal subjects. Eur Respir J 19(2):257–266
102. Zhou B et al (2005) Thymic stromal lymphopoietin as a key initiator of allergic airway inflammation in mice. Nat Immunol 6(10):1047
103. He R, Geha RS (2010) Thymic stromal lymphopoietin. Ann N Y Acad Sci 1183:13
104. Verstraelen S et al (2008) Cell types involved in allergic asthma and their use in in vitro models to assess respiratory sensitization. Toxicol In Vitro 22(6):1419–1431
105. Bharadwaj AS, Bewtra AK, Agrawal DK (2007) Dendritic cells in allergic airway inflammation. Can J Physiol Pharmacol 85(7):686–699
106. Gaurav R, Agrawal DK (2013) Clinical view on the importance of dendritic cells in asthma. Expert Rev Clin Immunol 9(10):899–919
107. Schon-Hegrad MA et al (1991) Studies on the density, distribution, and surface phenotype of intraepithelial class II major histocompatibility complex antigen (Ia)-bearing dendritic cells (DC) in the conducting airways. J Exp Med 173(6):1345–1356
108. Sun-sang JS, Rose CE, Fu SM (2001) Intratracheal priming with ovalbumin-and ovalbumin 323–339 peptide-pulsed dendritic cells induces airway hyperresponsiveness, lung eosinophilia, goblet cell hyperplasia, and inflammation. J Immunol 166(2):1261–1271
109. Wills-Karp M (2000) Murine models of asthma in understanding immune dysregulation in human asthma. Immunopharmacology 48(3):263–268
110. Hammad H et al (2009) House dust mite allergen induces asthma via Toll-like receptor 4 triggering of airway structural cells. Nat Med 15(4):410
111. van Rijt LS et al (2002) Allergen-induced accumulation of airway dendritic cells is supported by an increase in CD31hiLy-6Cneg bone marrow precursors in a mouse model of asthma. Blood 100(10):3663–3671
112. Lambrecht BN et al (1999) Allergen-induced changes in bone-marrow progenitor and airway dendritic cells in sensitized rats. Am J Respir Cell Mol Biol 20(6):1165–1174
113. Gregory LG, Lloyd CM (2011) Orchestrating house dust mite-associated allergy in the lung. Trends Immunol 32(9):402–411
114. Wills-Karp M (2010) Allergen-specific pattern recognition receptor pathways. Curr Opin Immunol 22(6):777–782
115. Penna G et al (2002) Differential migration behavior and chemokine production by myeloid and plasmacytoid dendritic cells. Hum Immunol 63(12):1164–1171
116. Hammad H et al (2003) Monocyte-derived dendritic cells exposed to Der p 1 allergen enhance the recruitment of Th2 cells: major involvement of the chemokines TARC\CCL17 and MDC \CCL22. Eur Cytokine Netw 14(4):219–228
117. Kawakami T, Galli SJ (2002) Regulation of mast-cell and basophil function and survival by IgE. Nat Rev Immunol 2(10):773
118. Metcalfe DD, Baram D, Mekori YA (1997) Mast cells. Physiol Rev 77:10331079
119. Venkatesha RT et al (2005) Distinct regulation of C3a-induced MCP-1/CCL2 and RANTES/CCL5 production in human mast cells by extracellular signal regulated kinase and PI3 kinase. Mol Immunol 42(5):581–587
120. Renauld J-C (2001) New insights into the role of cytokines in asthma. J Clin Pathol 54 (8):577–589
121. Barnes PJ (2017) Cellular and molecular mechanisms of asthma and COPD. Clin Sci 131 (13):1541–1558
122. Bradding P, Walls AF, Holgate ST (2006) The role of the mast cell in the pathophysiology of asthma. J Allergy Clin Immunol 117(6):1277–1284
123. Louahed J et al (2000) Interleukin-9 upregulates mucus expression in the airways. Am J Respir Cell Mol Biol 22(6):649–656
124. Ammit AJ et al (1997) Mast cell numbers are increased in the smooth muscle of human sensitized isolated bronchi. Am J Respir Crit Care Med 155(3):1123–1129

125. Carroll N, Mutavdzic S, James A (2002) Distribution and degranulation of airway mast cells in normal and asthmatic subjects. Eur Respir J 19(5):879–885
126. Chang TW et al (1990) Monoclonal antibodies specific for human IgE-producing B cells: a potential therapeutic for IgE-mediated allergic diseases. Bio/Technology 8(2):122
127. MacGlashan DW et al (1997) Down-regulation of Fc (epsilon) RI expression on human basophils during in vivo treatment of atopic patients with anti-IgE antibody. J Immunol 158 (3):1438–1445
128. Hart PH (2001) Regulation of the inflammatory response in asthma by mast cell products. Immunol Cell Biol 79(2):149–153
129. Holsapple MP et al (2005) Assessing the potential to induce respiratory hypersensitivity. Toxicol Sci 91(1):4–13
130. Schweitzer-Stenner R, Pecht I (2005) Cutting edge: death of a dogma or enforcing the artificial: monomeric IgE binding may initiate mast cell response by inducing its receptor aggregation. J Immunol 174(8):4461–4464
131. Kalesnikoff J et al (2001) Monomeric IgE stimulates signaling pathways in mast cells that lead to cytokine production and cell survival. Immunity 14(6):801–811
132. Balzar S et al (2005) Relationship of small airway chymase-positive mast cells and lung function in severe asthma. Am J Respir Crit Care Med 171(5):431–439
133. Kay AB, Klion AD (2004) Anti-interleukin-5 therapy for asthma and hypereosinophilic syndrome. Immunol Allergy Clin 24(4):645–666
134. Possa SS et al (2013) Eosinophilic inflammation in allergic asthma. Front Pharmacol 4:46
135. Jacobsen EA et al (2011) Eosinophils regulate dendritic cells and Th2 pulmonary immune responses following allergen provocation. J Immunol 187(11):6059–6068
136. Bousquet J et al (1990) Eosinophilic inflammation in asthma. N Engl J Med 323 (15):1033–1039
137. Price DB et al (2015) Blood eosinophil count and prospective annual asthma disease burden: a UK cohort study. Lancet Respir Med 3(11):849–858
138. Kita H (2011) Eosinophils: multifaceted biological properties and roles in health and disease. Immunol Rev 242(1):161–177
139. Schleich FN et al (2014) Importance of concomitant local and systemic eosinophilia in uncontrolled asthma. Eur Respir J 44(1):97–108
140. Roufosse F (2018) Targeting the interleukin-5 pathway for treatment of eosinophilic conditions other than asthma. Front Med 5:49
141. Vignola AM, Kips J, Bousquet J (2000) Tissue remodeling as a feature of persistent asthma. J Allergy Clin Immunol 105(6):1041–1053
142. Hendeles L, Asmus M, Chesrown S (2004) Evaluation of cytokine modulators for asthma. Paediatr Respir Rev 5:S107–S112
143. Lemanske RF Jr, Busse WW (2010) Asthma: clinical expression and molecular mechanisms. J Allergy Clin Immunol 125(2):S95–S102
144. Miyake K, Karasuyama H (2017) Emerging roles of basophils in allergic inflammation. Allergol Int 66(3):382–391
145. Wedemeyer J, Tsai M, Galli SJ (2000) Roles of mast cells and basophils in innate and acquired immunity. Curr Opin Immunol 12(6):624–631
146. Siracusa MC et al (2013) Basophils and allergic inflammation. J Allergy Clin Immunol 132 (4):789–801
147. Di C et al (2015) Basophil-associated OX40 ligand participates in the initiation of Th2 responses during airway inflammation. J Biol Chem 290(20):12523–12536
148. Rayees S et al (2015) Therapeutic effects of R8, a semi-synthetic analogue of Vasicine, on murine model of allergic airway inflammation via STAT6 inhibition. Int Immunopharmacol 26(1):246–256
149. Marone G, Triggiani M, de Paulis A (2005) Mast cells and basophils: friends as well as foes in bronchial asthma? Trends Immunol 26(1):25–31

150. Perrigoue JG et al (2009) MHC class II-dependent basophil–CD4+ T cell interactions promote TH2 cytokine-dependent immunity. Nat Immunol 10(7):697
151. Sokol CL et al (2009) Basophils function as antigen-presenting cells for an allergen-induced T helper type 2 response. Nat Immunol 10(7):713
152. Yoshimoto T et al (2009) Basophils contribute to TH2-IgE responses in vivo via IL-4 production and presentation of peptide–MHC class II complexes to CD4+ T cells. Nat Immunol 10(7):706
153. Douwes J et al (2002) Non-eosinophilic asthma: importance and possible mechanisms. Thorax 57(7):643–648
154. Ciepiela O, Ostafin M, Demkow U (2015) Neutrophils in asthma—a review. Respir Physiol Neurobiol 209:13–16
155. Radeau T et al (1990) Enhanced arachidonic acid metabolism and human neutrophil migration in asthma. Prostaglandins Leukot Essent Fat Acids 41(2):131–138
156. Wenzel SE et al (1997) Bronchoscopic evaluation of severe asthma: persistent inflammation associated with high dose glucocorticoids. Am J Respir Crit Care Med 156(3):737–743
157. Shaw DE et al (2007) Association between neutrophilic airway inflammation and airflow limitation in adults with asthma. Chest 132(6):1871–1875
158. Smit JJ, Lukacs NW (2006) A closer look at chemokines and their role in asthmatic responses. Eur J Pharmacol 533(1–3):277–288
159. Arjomandi M et al (2005) Repeated exposure to ozone increases alveolar macrophage recruitment into asthmatic airways. Am J Respir Crit Care Med 172(4):427–432
160. Gordon S, Martinez FO (2010) Alternative activation of macrophages: mechanism and functions. Immunity 32(5):593–604
161. Leung T et al (2004) Increased macrophage-derived chemokine in exhaled breath condensate and plasma from children with asthma. Clin Exp Allergy 34(5):786–791
162. Mautino G et al (1999) Increased expression of tissue inhibitor of metalloproteinase-1 and loss of correlation with matrix metalloproteinase-9 by macrophages in asthma. Lab Invest 79 (1):39–47
163. Moon K-A et al (2007) Allergen-induced CD11b+ CD11cint CCR3+ macrophages in the lung promote eosinophilic airway inflammation in a mouse asthma model. Int Immunol 19 (12):1371–1381
164. Balhara J, Gounni A (2012) The alveolar macrophages in asthma: a double-edged sword. Mucosal Immunol 5(6):605
165. Hoshi H et al (1995) IL-5, IL-8 and GM-CSF immunostaining of sputum cells in bronchial asthma and chronic bronchitis. Clin Exp Allergy 25(8):720–728
166. Ackerman V et al (1994) Detection of cytokines and their cell sources in bronchial biopsy specimens from asthmatic patients: relationship to atopic status, symptoms, and level of airway hyperresponsiveness. Chest 105(3):687–696
167. Chanez P et al (1994) Modulation by interleukin-4 of cytokine release from mononuclear phagocytes in asthma. J Allergy Clin Immunol 94(6):997–1005
168. Gosset P et al (1992) Tumor necrosis factor alpha and interleukin-6 production by human mononuclear phagocytes from allergic asthmatics after IgE-dependent stimulation. Am Rev Respir Dis 146:768–768
169. Gosset P et al (1999) Production of chemokines and proinflammatory and antiinflammatory cytokines by human alveolar macrophages activated by IgE receptors. J Allergy Clin Immunol 103(2):289–297
170. Wiest M et al (2018) Clinical implications of CD4+ T cell subsets in adult atopic asthma patients. Allergy Asthma Clin Immunol 14(1):7
171. Tang C et al (1997) IL-5 production by bronchoalveolar lavage and peripheral blood mononuclear cells in asthma and atopy. Eur Respir J 10(3):624–632
172. Park CS et al (1996) Interleukin-4 and low-affinity receptor for IgE on B cells in peripheral blood of patients with atopic bronchial asthma. J Allergy Clin Immunol 97(5):1121–1128

173. Kenyon NJ, Kelly EA, Jarjour NN (2000) Enhanced cytokine generation by peripheral blood mononuclear cells in allergic and asthma subjects. Ann Allergy Asthma Immunol 85 (2):115–120
174. Tang C et al (1998) Alveolar macrophages from atopic asthmatics, but not atopic nonasthmatics, enhance interleukin-5 production by CD4+ T cells. Am J Respir Crit Care Med 157(4):1120–1126
175. Tang C et al (1999) Modulatory effects of alveolar macrophages on CD4+ T-cell IL-5 responses correlate with IL-1beta, IL-6, and IL-12 production. Eur Respir J 14(1):106–112
176. Kelly EAB et al (1997) The effect of segmental bronchoprovocation with allergen on airway lymphocyte function. Am J Respir Crit Care Med 156(5):1421–1428
177. Nakamura Y et al (1999) Gene expression of the GATA-3 transcription factor is increased in atopic asthma. J Allergy Clin Immunol 103(2):215–222
178. Taha R et al (2003) T helper type 2 cytokine receptors and associated transcription factors GATA-3, c-MAF, and signal transducer and activator of transcription factor-6 in induced sputum of atopic asthmatic patients. Chest 123(6):2074–2082
179. Takeda K et al (2009) Vaccine-induced CD8+ T cell-dependent suppression of airway hyperresponsiveness and inflammation. J Immunol 183(1):181–190
180. Ying S et al (1997) Expression of IL-4 and IL-5 mRNA and protein product by CD4+ and CD8 + T cells, eosinophils, and mast cells in bronchial biopsies obtained from atopic and nonatopic (intrinsic) asthmatics. J Immunol 158(7):3539–3544
181. Gelfand EW et al (2017) Spectrum of T-lymphocyte activities regulating allergic lung inflammation. Immunol Rev 278(1):63–86
182. Hamelmann E et al (1996) Requirement for CD8+ T cells in the development of airway hyperresponsiveness in a marine model of airway sensitization. J Exp Med 183(4):1719–1729
183. Tsitsiou E et al (2012) Transcriptome analysis shows activation of circulating CD8+ T cells in patients with severe asthma. J Allergy Clin Immunol 129(1):95–103
184. Hilvering B et al (2018) Synergistic activation of pro-inflammatory type-2 CD8+ T lymphocytes by lipid mediators in severe eosinophilic asthma. Mucosal Immunol 11(5):1408
185. Ano S et al (2013) Transcription factors GATA-3 and RORγt are important for determining the phenotype of allergic airway inflammation in a murine model of asthma. J Immunol 190 (3):1056–1065
186. Larché M, Robinson DS, Kay AB (2003) The role of T lymphocytes in the pathogenesis of asthma. J Allergy Clin Immunol 111(3):450–463
187. Ngoc LP et al (2005) Cytokines, allergy, and asthma. Curr Opin Allergy Clin Immunol 5 (2):161–166
188. Barnes PJ, Adcock I (1998) Transcription factors and asthma. Eur Respir J 12(1):221–234
189. Cousins DJ, McDonald J, Lee TH (2008) Therapeutic approaches for control of transcription factors in allergic disease. J Allergy Clin Immunol 121(4):803–809
190. Barnes PJ, Karin M (1997) Nuclear factor-κB—a pivotal transcription factor in chronic inflammatory diseases. N Engl J Med 336(15):1066–1071
191. Bureau F et al (2000) Mechanisms of persistent NF-κB activity in the bronchi of an animal model of asthma. J Immunol 165(10):5822–5830
192. Gagliardo R et al (2003) Persistent activation of nuclear factor-κB signaling pathway in severe uncontrolled asthma. Am J Respir Crit Care Med 168(10):1190–1198
193. Hart LA et al (1998) Activation and localization of transcription factor, nuclear factor-κB, in asthma. Am J Respir Crit Care Med 158(5):1585–1592
194. Poynter ME, Irvin CG, Janssen-Heininger YM (2002) Rapid activation of nuclear factor-κB in airway epithelium in a murine model of allergic airway inflammation. Am J Pathol 160 (4):1325–1334
195. Yang L et al (1998) Essential role of nuclear factor κB in the induction of eosinophilia in allergic airway inflammation. J Exp Med 188(9):1739–1750
196. Donovan CE et al (1999) NF-κB/Rel transcription factors: c-Rel promotes airway hyperresponsiveness and allergic pulmonary inflammation. J Immunol 163(12):6827–6833

197. Das J et al (2001) A critical role for NF-κB in GATA3 expression and T H 2 differentiation in allergic airway inflammation. Nat Immunol 2(1):45
198. Choi I-W et al (2004) Administration of antisense phosphorothioate oligonucleotide to the p65 subunit of NF-κB inhibits established asthmatic reaction in mice. Int Immunopharmacol 4 (14):1817–1828
199. Rahman I (2005) Redox signaling in the lungs. Antioxid Redox Signal 7(1–2):1–5
200. Yuan F et al (2019) JAX2, an ethanol extract of Hyssopus cuspidatus Boriss, can prevent bronchial asthma by inhibiting MAPK/NF-κB inflammatory signaling. Phytomedicine 57:305–314
201. Kaplan MH, Grusby MJ (1998) Regulation of T helper cell differentiation by STAT molecules. J Leukoc Biol 64(1):2–5
202. Palmer-Crocker RL, Hughes C, Pober JS (1996) IL-4 and IL-13 activate the JAK2 tyrosine kinase and Stat6 in cultured human vascular endothelial cells through a common pathway that does not involve the gamma c chain. J Clin Invest 98(3):604–609
203. Ray A, Cohn L (1999) Th2 cells and GATA-3 in asthma: new insights into the regulation of airway inflammation. J Clin Invest 104(8):985–993
204. Kaplan MH et al (1996) Stat6 is required for mediating responses to IL-4 and for the development of Th2 cells. Immunity 4(3):313–319
205. Shimoda K et al (1996) Lack of IL-4-induced Th2 response and IgE class switching in mice with disrupted State6 gene. Nature 380(6575):630
206. Takeda K et al (1996) Essential role of Stat6 in IL-4 signalling. Nature 380(6575):627
207. Yokozeki H et al (2000) Signal transducer and activator of transcription 6 is essential in the induction of contact hypersensitivity. J Exp Med 191(6):995–1004
208. Yokozeki H et al (2004) In vivo transfection of a cis element 'decoy' against signal transducers and activators of transcription 6 (STAT6)-binding site ameliorates IgE-mediated late-phase reaction in an atopic dermatitis mouse model. Gene Ther 11(24):1753
209. Hill S et al (1999) Homologous human and murine antisense oligonucleotides targeting Stat6: functional effects on germline C ε transcript. Am J Respir Cell Mol Biol 21(6):728–737
210. Peng Q, Matsuda T, Hirst SJ (2004) Signaling pathways regulating interleukin-13-stimulated chemokine release from airway smooth muscle. Am J Respir Crit Care Med 169(5):596–603
211. Chiba Y, Todoroki M, Misawa M (2009) Activation of signal transducer and activator of transcription factor 1 by interleukins-13 and -4 in cultured human bronchial smooth muscle cells. J Smooth Muscle Res 45(6):279–288
212. Darcan-Nicolaisen Y et al (2009) Small interfering RNA against transcription factor STAT6 inhibits allergic airway inflammation and hyperreactivity in mice. J Immunol 182 (12):7501–7508
213. Ho I et al (1991) Human GATA-3: a lineage-restricted transcription factor that regulates the expression of the T cell receptor alpha gene. EMBO J 10(5):1187–1192
214. Ansel KM et al (2006) Regulation of Th2 differentiation and Il4 locus accessibility. Annu Rev Immunol 24:607–656
215. Santangelo S et al (2002) DNA methylation changes at human Th2 cytokine genes coincide with DNase I hypersensitive site formation during CD4+ T cell differentiation. J Immunol 169 (4):1893–1903
216. Rayees S et al (2014) Linking GATA-3 and interleukin-13: implications in asthma. Inflamm Res 63(4):255–265
217. Lee HJ et al (2000) GATA-3 induces T helper cell type 2 (Th2) cytokine expression and chromatin remodeling in committed Th1 cells. J Exp Med 192(1):105–116
218. Sundrud MS et al (2003) Genetic reprogramming of primary human T cells reveals functional plasticity in Th cell differentiation. J Immunol 171(7):3542–3549
219. Zhang D-H et al (1999) Inhibition of allergic inflammation in a murine model of asthma by expression of a dominant-negative mutant of GATA-3. Immunity 11(4):473–482
220. Kiwamoto T et al (2006) Transcription factors T-bet and GATA-3 regulate development of airway remodeling. Am J Respir Crit Care Med 174(2):142–151

221. Yamashita N et al (2006) Involvement of GATA-3-dependent Th2 lymphocyte activation in airway hyperresponsiveness. Am J Phys Lung Cell Mol Phys 290(6):L1045–L1051
222. Lee C-C, Huang H-Y, Chiang B-L (2008) Lentiviral-mediated GATA-3 RNAi decreases allergic airway inflammation and hyperresponsiveness. Mol Ther 16(1):60–65
223. Rayees S et al (2014) Anti-asthmatic activity of azepino [2, 1-b] quinazolones, synthetic analogues of vasicine, an alkaloid from Adhatoda vasica. Med Chem Res 23(9):4269–4279
224. Hogan PG et al (2003) Transcriptional regulation by calcium, calcineurin, and NFAT. Genes Dev 17(18):2205–2232
225. Crabtree GR, Olson EN (2002) NFAT signaling: choreographing the social lives of cells. Cell 109(2):S67–S79
226. Macian F (2005) NFAT proteins: key regulators of T-cell development and function. Nat Rev Immunol 5(6):472
227. Peng SL et al (2001) NFATc1 and NFATc2 together control both T and B cell activation and differentiation. Immunity 14(1):13–20
228. Jia X et al (2014) Activation of TRPV1 mediates thymic stromal lymphopoietin release via the Ca^{2+}/NFAT pathway in airway epithelial cells. FEBS Lett 588(17):3047–3054
229. Jairaman A et al (2015) Store-operated Ca^{2+} release-activated Ca^{2+} channels regulate PAR2-activated Ca^{2+} signaling and cytokine production in airway epithelial cells. J Immunol 195 (5):2122–2133
230. Jairaman A et al (2016) Allergens stimulate store-operated calcium entry and cytokine production in airway epithelial cells. Sci Rep 6:32311
231. Global Initiative for Asthma (2018) GINA report, global strategy for asthma management and prevention. Global Initiative for Asthma, Fontana, WI
232. Bateman ED et al (2004) Can guideline-defined asthma control be achieved? The Gaining Optimal Asthma ControL study. Am J Respir Crit Care Med 170(8):836–844
233. Reddel HK et al (2019) GINA 2019: a fundamental change in asthma management: treatment of asthma with short-acting bronchodilators alone is no longer recommended for adults and adolescents. Eur Respir J 53(6)
234. Urbano FL (2008) Review of the NAEPP 2007 Expert Panel Report (EPR-3) on asthma diagnosis and treatment guidelines. J Manag Care Pharm 14(1):41–49
235. Zahran HS et al (2017) Long-term control medication use and asthma control status among children and adults with asthma. J Asthma 54(10):1065–1072
236. National Asthma Education and Prevention Program (2007) Expert Panel Report 3 (EPR-3): guidelines for the diagnosis and management of asthma-summary report 2007. J Allergy Clin Immunol 120(5 Suppl):S94
237. Diver S, Russell R, Brightling C (2018) New and emerging drug treatments for severe asthma. Clin Exp Allergy 48(3):241–252
238. Weatherall M et al (2009) Dose–response relationship of inhaled corticosteroids and cataracts: a systematic review and meta-analysis. Respirology 14(7):983–990
239. Schofield ML (2014) Asthma pharmacotherapy. Otolaryngol Clin N Am 47(1):55–64
240. Matsuse H, Kohno S (2014) Leukotriene receptor antagonists pranlukast and montelukast for treating asthma. Expert Opin Pharmacother 15(3):353–363
241. National Asthma Education and Prevention Program (2003) Expert panel report: guidelines for the diagnosis and management of asthma: update on selected topics, 2002. US Department of Health and Human Services, Public Health Service, National Institutes of Health
242. Ducharme F, di Salvio F (2004) Anti-leukotriene agents compared to inhaled corticosteroids in the management of recurrent and/or chronic asthma in adults and children. Cochrane Database Syst Rev (1)
243. Dahlén S-E et al (2002) Improvement of aspirin-intolerant asthma by montelukast, a leukotriene antagonist: a randomized, double-blind, placebo-controlled trial. Am J Respir Crit Care Med 165(1):9–14
244. Barnes PJ (2008) Drugs for airway disease. Medicine 36(4):181–190
245. Rees J (2006) Asthma control in adults. BMJ 332(7544):767–771

246. Scullion J (2010) Prescribing beta-agonists for respiratory disease. Independent Nurse
247. Buhl R, Hamelmann E (2019) Future perspectives of anticholinergics for the treatment of asthma in adults and children. Ther Clin Risk Manag 15:473
248. Hamelmann E (2018) Long-acting muscarinic antagonists for the treatment of asthma in children—a new kid in town. Allergo J 27(7):24–31
249. Kerstjens HA et al (2016) Tiotropium improves lung function, exacerbation rate, and asthma control, independent of baseline characteristics including age, degree of airway obstruction, and allergic status. Respir Med 117:198–206
250. Kang JY et al (2012) Effect of tiotropium bromide on airway remodeling in a chronic asthma model. Ann Allergy Asthma Immunol 109(1):29–35
251. Ohta S et al (2010) Effect of tiotropium bromide on airway inflammation and remodelling in a mouse model of asthma. Clin Exp Allergy 40(8):1266–1275
252. Bosnjak B et al (2014) Tiotropium bromide inhibits relapsing allergic asthma in BALB/c mice. Pulm Pharmacol Ther 27(1):44–51
253. Food and Drug Administration (2018) Prescribing information for Spiriva® Respimat® (tiotropium bromide) inhalation spray, for oral inhalation
254. Ingelheim B (2018) Asthma: expanded indication for SPIRIVA® Respimat® for people 6 years and older
255. Moulton BC, Fryer AD (2011) Muscarinic receptor antagonists, from folklore to pharmacology; finding drugs that actually work in asthma and COPD. Br J Pharmacol 163(1):44–52
256. Ward M et al (1981) Ipratropium bromide in acute asthma. Br Med J (Clin Res Ed) 282 (6264):598–600
257. Donohue JF et al (2016) Efficacy and safety of ipratropium bromide/albuterol compared with albuterol in patients with moderate-to-severe asthma: a randomized controlled trial. BMC Pulm Med 16(1):65
258. Lougheed MD et al (2010) Canadian Thoracic Society Asthma Management Continuum–2010 Consensus Summary for children six years of age and over, and adults. Can Respir J 17 (1):15–24
259. Jolobe O (1984) Asthma vs. non-specific reversible airflow obstruction: clinical features and responsiveness to anticholinergic drugs. Respiration 45(3):237–242
260. Lee TA et al (2008) Risk for death associated with medications for recently diagnosed chronic obstructive pulmonary disease. Ann Intern Med 149(6):380–390
261. Ogale SS et al (2010) Cardiovascular events associated with ipratropium bromide in COPD. Chest 137(1):13–19
262. Buhl R (2005) Anti-IgE antibodies for the treatment of asthma. Curr Opin Pulm Med 11 (1):27–34
263. Fahy J (2000) New and exploratory therapeutic agents for asthma: lung biology in health and disease. Marcel Dekker, Inc., New York, NY
264. Yeadon M, Diamant Z (1999) New and exploratory therapeutic agents for asthma, vol 139. CRC Press, Boca Raton
265. D'Amato G, Oldani V, Donner C (2002) Treating atopic asthma with the anti-IgE monoclonal antibody. Monaldi Arch Chest Dis 57(2):117–119
266. Riccio A et al (2012) Omalizumab modulates bronchial reticular basement membrane thickness and eosinophil infiltration in severe persistent allergic asthma patients. Int J Immunopathol Pharmacol 25(2):475–484
267. Hoshino M, Ohtawa J (2012) Effects of adding omalizumab, an anti-immunoglobulin E antibody, on airway wall thickening in asthma. Respiration 83(6):520–528
268. D'Amato G et al (2014) Treating severe allergic asthma with anti-IgE monoclonal antibody (omalizumab): a review. Multidiscip Respir Med 9(1):23
269. Pelaia G et al (2011) Update on optimal use of omalizumab in management of asthma. J Asthma Allergy 4:49

270. National Asthma Education and Prevention Program (2002) Expert Panel Report: guidelines for the diagnosis and management of asthma update on selected topics—2002. J Allergy Clin Immunol 110(5 Suppl):S141
271. Leung K et al (1988) Effects of sodium cromoglycate and nedocromil sodium on histamine secretion from human lung mast cells. Thorax 43(10):756–761
272. Netzer NC et al (2012) The actual role of sodium cromoglycate in the treatment of asthma—a critical review. Sleep Breath 16(4):1027–1032

Cystic Fibrosis: Biology and Therapeutics

3

Pritt Verma, Vishal Kumar Vishwakarma, Shravan Kumar Paswan, Ch. V. Rao, and Sajal Srivastava

Abstract

Cystic fibrosis could be a common life-bound autosomal recessive hereditary condition, with highest occurrence in Europe, North America, and Australia. The root of illness is mutation of a gene that encodes a chloride-conducting transmembrane channel known as the cystic fibrosis transmembrane conductance regulator (CFTR) that regulates anion transfer and mucociliary clearance within the airways. Operational failure of CFTR ends up in mucus withholding and chronic contagion, followed by local airway swelling that is harmful to the lungs. CFTR operational impairment principally affects epithelial cells, though there is proof of a function in immune cells. Cystic fibrosis influences numerous body systems, and morbidity and mortality are typically due to bronchiectasis, tiny airways obstacle, and progressive respiratory abnormality. Necessary comorbidities due to epithelial cell operational impairment occur within the pancreas (malassimilation), liver (biliary cirrhosis), sweat glands (heat shock), and vas deferens (sterility). The progress and delivery of medication that recover the clearance of mucus from the lungs and treat the ensuing infection, together with rectification of pancreatic insufficiency and malnutrition via multidisciplinary requisites, have resulted in noteworthy enhancements of life and clinical conclusion in patients with cystic fibrosis. Inventive and transformational treatments that aim on the fundamental defect in cystic fibrosis have currently been grown and are useful in lung surgery and dropping pulmonary

P. Verma (✉) · S. K. Paswan · C. V. Rao
Pharmacology Division, CSIR-National Botanical Research Institute, Lucknow, Uttar Pradesh, India
e-mail: preetverma06@gmail.com

V. K. Vishwakarma
Department of Pharmacology, All India Institute of Medical Sciences (AIIMS), New Delhi, India

S. Srivastava
Amity Institute of Pharmacy, Amity University Uttar Pradesh, Lucknow, Uttar Pradesh, India

S. Rayees et al. (eds.), *Chronic Lung Diseases*,
https://doi.org/10.1007/978-981-15-3734-9_3

exacerbations. Advance petite molecule and gene-based treatment are being developed to revive CFTR operation; these remedies pledge to transform illness and enhance the lives of individuals with cystic fibrosis disease.

Keywords

Cystic fibrosis · CFTR · Bronchiectasis · Ivacaftor · Lumacaftor · Orkambi

3.1 Introduction

3.1.1 About the Disease

Cystic fibrosis (CF) respiratory organ malady is characterized by early organization and infection of the airways. Though structural changes within the CF airways will be ascertained at birth in each human and therefore the CF pig, modest inflammation is ascertained [1–3]. However, infection happens terribly apace and therefore the inflammatory response to pathogens is harsh [4]. Free and leap airway neutrophil elastase is detected terribly early in CF infants and predicts the event of bronchiectasis later in life [5]. No further respiratory organ malady is understood to induce such an untimely, persistent, and intense inflammatory method as seen within the CF airway. People with CF conjointly suffer from an extreme general inflammation characterized by inflated serum acute-phase reactants, high antibody titers to various exogenous and endogenous antigens, and an elevated occurrence of ileum inflammation with Crohn's malady, instant hypersensitivity, and heightened Th2 responses [6, 7].

3.1.2 Epidemiology

The global occurrence and dominance of CF show important geographical inconsistency, as illustrated by the detection rates seen globally. Within the USA, the incidence of CF is reported to be 1 in each 3500 births [8]. Though a better incidence is noted in European nations at a rate of 1 in each of 2000–3000 births, in Africa and Asia, though CF is sternly beneath diagnosed, proof indicates that the prevalence of CF is low down to atypical [8, 9].

3.1.3 Causes

CF is caused by a severe functional scarcity of the cystic fibrosis transmembrane conductance regulator (CFTR) protein [10]. CFTR is mostly expressed within the apex membranes of epithelial cells that line the cylindrical structures of tissues that secrete fluids typically made in mucous secretion and different proteins. The airways are amid the tissues with the utmost expression of CFTR. The scarcity of functional

CFTR causes scarce cAMP-dependent chloride and hydrogen carbonate secretion into airway secretions. Consequently, mucins are bound to the bronchial apex surfaces, and airway surface fluid pH scale is weakened [11].

3.2 Pathophysiology

The types of complications in patients with CF vary depending on the extent of mutation of CFTR. Also, some patients do not feel the pathological changes altogether as the system is typically affected with CF.

3.2.1 Biology of Disease

3.2.1.1 Respiratory System

Typically, critically sick patients who have CF feel acute respiratory failure owing to pneumonia or acute hemoptysis. The foremost common infecting organisms in patients with CF which have pneumonia include *Staphylococcus aureus*, *Haemophilus influenzae*, and *Pseudomonas aeruginosa*. Noteworthy, patients with CF additionally tend to own nasal polyps that may trigger sinus infections. Thus, these patients may have longer and completely special antibiotic treatments than do patients who have pneumonia exclusively. It is hypothesized that the pH scale level within the cells of patients with cystic fibrosis differs from the extent in patients devoid of the disease. This distinction results in magnified numbers of asialoGM1 molecules that are receptors intended for bacterial respiratory organisms, and thereby ends up in magnified binding of *P. aeruginosa* and *S. aureus*. The decline within the quantity of CFTR to bind with the bacteria results in colonization of the airways [12]. In a very few patients with CF who have pneumonia, the pneumonia is because of *Burkholderia cepacia* (previously referred to as *Pseudomonas cepacia*), which is extremely immune to most antibiotics.

As obstacle of the airway will amplify, it becomes harder for air to pass throughout exhalation. This condition results in enlargement of alveoli, wherever air lock happens and, over time, causes the barrel-shaped chest that is additionally general in patients with emphysema. Destruction of the pulmonary parenchyma results in magnified pulmonary blood pressure that, in turn, causes right-sided heart failure or core pulmonale.

Pulmonary performance testing may be a methodology that will be useful in establishing information that will assist in predicting deterioration in clinical standing in patients with CF [13]. One factor, forced expiratory volume in 1 s (FEV1), is usually used as an indicator of the worsening condition. The lower the FEV1, the effort of breathing increases; it is related with gas exchange [14]. The amplified work of breathing will embody any of the following: tachypnea, uneven breathing pattern, perspiration, spread nares, pursed lip breathing, intercostal muscle retractions, and use of retrofit muscles. Patients with lower FEV1 additionally tend to be in a very chronic state of acidosis and, similar to additional patients with chronic obstructive pulmonary disease, may have lower PaO_2 levels to trigger the hypoxic ventilatory force, though they still want adequate oxygenation. Association or enlargement of the last joints of the toes and fingers, which have no definite cause, additionally happens in patients with CF.

Typically, patients with CF have declined levels of interleukin-10, a cytokine that has anti-inflammatory properties, particularly within the lungs [15]. The drop off levels disposes the patients to severe lung inflammation subsequent to infection. Occasionally, the pulmonary inflammation persists and becomes a chronic inflammatory situation. Chronic inflammation will cause hypertrophy of the bronchial arteries and ultimately, hemoptysis. This critical condition is more worsened by coagulopathies usually caused by malabsorption of vitamin K and perennial use of some antibiotic. The manifestation of hemoptysis varies from blood-tinged bodily sputum to enormous hemorrhaging. It is thought that 5–7% of patients with CF truly have enormous hemoptysis [16].

Patients with CF, who have elevated levels of thick and firm mucus secretion in their airways, are usually admitted to the intensive care unit on account of flow of air limitation. The foremost severe respiratory signs and symptoms are because of the creation of elevated levels of thickened mucus secretion that cause inflammation and swelling and therefore barred airways. The obstruction causes consolidation that results in pneumonia and respiratory failure. Often, patients have elevated withholding of mucus secretion within the right upper lobe, which is indicated by proof of hyperinflation on chest radiographs [17].

Approximately 10% of patients with CF too have infection caused by the fungus *Aspergillus fumigatus*, which might cause allergic bronchopulmonary aspergillosis and end up in a dramatic enhancement in secretions and an ultimate downward twist in the lung task [18]. Patients with sinobronchial allergic zymosis and/or allergic bronchopulmonary mycosis have terribly thick secretions and are immune to antibiotics. The patients with allergic bronchopulmonary do not show any sign and symptoms of Cystic fibrosis before sinobronchial allergic mycosis. In addition to/or else allergic bronchopulmonary mycosis develops, however once tested are found to own mutation(s) within the CFTR factor [18–20]. In several patients, CF is misdiagnosed as celiac disorder, asthma, or chronic bronchitis [21].

3.2.1.2 Hematopoietic System

Patients with CF own iron-deficit anemia and usually have anemia as a results of chronic hemoptysis in addition to or else colonization of resistant *P. aeruginosa* [22]. Blood loss usually comes from the hypertrophied and tortuous bronchial arteries as an outcome of chronic inflammation [16]. *Pseudomonas aeruginosa*, an antibiotic-resistant bacteria within the lungs addition to/or else superior airways of patients with CF, steals iron from the host for its self-growth. Additionally, sputum and bronchial airway cleaning fluid of patients with CF who have *P. aeruginosa* infection include a high iron content [23].

3.2.1.3 Gastrointestinal System

Some gastrointestinal issues in patients with CF are due to the lack of pancreas to produce digestive enzymes to the bowel. As a result of the quantity of pancreatic enzymes discharge decline, the pancreas oozes thick mucus that obstructs the pancreatic ducts and therefore the number of enzymes that may be secreted becomes yet lesser. This alteration causes malassimilation of proteins and persuades absorption of the fat-soluble vitamins A, D, E, and K. The pancreatic enzyme supplements that various patients with CF take could spoil iron assimilation [22]. It is suggested that patients with CF take supplements and vitamins individually.

The distal fraction of the bowel is usually expanded and crammed with fecal content in patients with CF. This alteration is manifested as vomiting, abdominal distention, anorexia, pain within the right lower quadrant of the abdomen, and cramping with a decline or no modification in intestinal movements [23]. Distal intestinal obstruction syndrome (DIOS) may be a result of defective oozing of salt and water from the intestinal epithelium, a state that causes dehydration of the intestinal material.

Some patients with cystic fibrosis even have gastroesophageal reflux disease (GERD) because of hypersecretion of gastric acid and hyposecretion of bicarbonate [23]. Postural emptying will worsen GERD, as will the negative pressures generated by strong coughing. GERD will likewise worsen bronchial reactivity.

3.2.1.4 Endocrine System

About 13% of all patients having CF own cystic fibrosis-associated diabetes that is most frequently diagnosed once the patients are 30 years old. Studies signify that the evaluation of glycated hemoglobin (hemoglobin A_{1C}) does not seem to be a correct diagnostic assay for cystic fibrosis-associated diabetes; as a result, the turnover of red blood cells is more rapid in patients with cystic fibrosis than in patients with no cystic fibrosis [24]. The first downside in cystic fibrosis-associated diabetes is insulin deficit because of barrier of the pancreatic duct. Patients with cystic fibrosis-associated diabetes still need a high-energy diet that is contrary to the diet that others with diabetes mellitus should follow. Glucose metabolism is influenced by several reasons particular to CF, such as severe dehydration, administration of corticosteroids, malassimilation, repeated contamination, poor nutrition, amplified energy expenditure, slowed gastrointestinal travel time, and liver dysfunction [25].

3.2.1.5 Sweat Glands

On account of the declined levels of the protein CFTR, which assists to control salt in sweat, patients with CF will feel too much salt loss from extreme temperature or compared to tremendous work out. Several patients feel dehydration or high-temperature prostration manifested by sluggishness, weakness, and loss of hunger.

3.2.1.6 Reproductive System

Most men with CF are sterile; as a result, they do not have vas deferens or it is misshapen. Women have a tendency to be fertile; however, they usually need longer to become pregnant than do women devoid of CF. Mucus discharge plugs within the oviduct and thicker cervical mucus that lessen sperm movement are detected [23]. Puberty appears to be delayed for each men and women who have this problem.

3.2.2 Cell Type Involved

The lung is continuously exposed to both noxious and infectious agents, and a multi-tiered defense has evolved that is able to continuously cleanse airways without inciting a potentially harmful inflammatory response. The mucus clearance (MC) system appears to be paramount for airways defense and is the locus of defects that lead to genetic lung diseases such as CF and primary ciliary dyskinesia. Other important elements in this defense system include locally residing leukocytes (e.g., alveolar and airway macrophages), mucosal immunoglobulins, and secreted antimicrobial compounds (e.g., lysozyme and lactoferrin), all of which are available to neutralize microbes that escape the first line of defense, that is, mechanical MC. A normally functioning MC apparatus requires the coordinated activities of mucus secretion, salt and water transport, and ciliary beating. Mucus secretion creates a protective blanket that efficiently binds inhaled particles via its panoply of carbohydrate epitopes, where they become entrapped via turbulent flow. The mucus layer, which floats on top of a less viscous and physically distinct liquid layer, is propelled cephalad by a combination of coordinated cilia beating and airflow/cough. The underlying liquid layer, often referred to as the "sol" or "periciliary liquid" layer (PCL), is itself quite complex and specially structured to provide a low resistance environment for ciliary beating while allowing efficient mechanical coupling between the tips of cilia and the mucus layer.

3.2.3 Transcription Regulation

To understand the pathophysiology of CF, one of the approaches is to discover the CFTR expression pattern in different tissue surveys. CFTR is found to be expressed in the epithelial cells of a variety of tissues and organs, whose functions are significantly affected in CF patients: lung and trachea, pancreas, liver, intestines, and sweat glands. Low levels of CFTR transcripts can be found in kidney, uterus, ovary, thyroid, and even higher levels in salivary gland and bladder, but the epithelial cell function is not seriously compromised in tissues and organs of CF patients. It is possible that there is sufficient compensation of the missing function by other ion transporters. It is of interest to note that the low levels of CFTR expression in these tissues are driven off an alternative promoter.

The majority of CFTR transcripts are driven from the key promoter, described in the previous section. However, although the canonical transcripts are found in cells with high CFTR expression, alternative transcription start sites are apparently used in cell lines with low expression levels. CFTR transcripts from even more distant transcription start sites between −868 and −794 can be found in CFPAC and T84 cell lines.

The immediate promoter region has also been characterized by consensus binding sites for several transcription factors: CTCF, AP-1, SP1, GRE, CRE, C/EBP, and Y-box proteins. DNase I hypersensitive site (DHS) mapping has been used to map various putative enhancer sequences within the CFTR intragenic regions. Presumably, multiple transcription factors can bind to chromatin at these sequences, opening the DNA and extending the physical interactions with the promoter, thereby affecting transcription. HNF1α binding sites, indicative of putative enhancer elements, can be found in multiple locations inside introns 10, 17a, and 20; it has been shown that RNAi-mediated inhibition of the HNF1α could lead to reduction of CFTR expression. Additional enhancer elements have been located in introns 1 and 11, and HNF1α and p300 are involved in the regulation of CFTR expression.

3.3 Current Treatment

The purpose of treatment mainly consists of the following:

3.3.1 Respiratory System

Stopping and regulating lung infections: Antibiotics are given. This primarily carries with it inhaled varieties of azithromycin, tobramycin, aztreonam and levofloxacin. Alternative antibiotics suggested are cipro, cephalexin, larotid, and doxycycline depending on the sensitivity patterns [26, 27].

Management of airway inflammation: NSAIDs, breathe in and systemic steroids and cromolyn [28].

Reducing viscoelasticity and eliminating thick, sticky mucus discharge from the lungs and expanding the airways: breathe in β-agonists with dampened oxygen; a 3–6% hypertonic saline solution and dornase alfa are suggested [29–31].

Additionally, workout and physiotherapy together with positive expiratory pressure (PEP) tool or an elevated occurrence chest wall swinging device (a percussion vest) is suggested [32].

3.3.2 Gastrointestinal Tract

Avoid or taking care of intestinal obstruction: oral rehydration and osmotic laxatives (unfinished obstruction) and hyperosmolar contrast enemas (total DIOS). An unbiased electrolyte bowel-cleaning solution or enema including diatrizoate meglumine and diatrizoate sodium, depending on vomiting condition [33]. To forestall repetition, regular administration of oral polythene glycol 3350 is also given for 6 months to 1 year.

Pancreatic insufficiency: pancreatic enzyme replacement therapy (PERT) containing multiple mixture of proteases, lipases, and amylases [34].

3.3.3 Nutrition and Electrolyte

Providing relevant nutrition and put off dehydration: A high-calorie-fat diet, add-on of vitamins ADEK, and minerals as well as fluoride and zinc are suggested. Furthermore, sodium chloride add-on is given customized to patient's age and environmental conditions [35].

In the earlier period, Denufosol, an agonist of P2Y2 receptors was attempted in CF patients; however, it was eventually unsuccessful subsequent to early promising outcome.

3.3.4 Current and Future Medicinal Products

The present and upcoming therapeutic objects are primarily focused on exact structural and purposeful anomaly of CFTR protein.

3.3.4.1 CFTR Modulators

A new cluster of medicine, known as CFTR modulators, is offered that is ready to correct the essential defect in CF, that is, CFTR protein itself; however, the specific mechanism is not absolutely clarified.

3.3.4.2 Ivacaftor

Developed by vertex pharmaceuticals and permitted by FDA in 2012 for kids ≥6 years having rare mutation, G551D (class III), ivacaftor (Kalydeco) [36] was the primary doing-well medication to fix the malfunctioning protein and was tried to be terribly effective in two massive multicentric trials, STRIVE and ENVISION [37, 38]. Marked improvements in FEV1, weight and quality of life were ascertained. Currently, the FDA has enlarged its use in alternative mutations and additionally kids aged 2–5 years supported the results of KIWI trial [39]. In addition, a phase IV clinical trials study (GOAL) additionally reported development in FEV1 and FVC, BMI, quality of life and bated sweat chloride concentration in patients carrying a minimum of one G551D allele. Over 72% patients during this trial additionally carried F508del as second allele [40]. The G551D mutation causes the channel to act as sort of a secured gate, avoiding the transconductance of chloride and fluid. The site of channel is correct; however, the performance is impaired. Ivacaftor will increase the time of channel in an open state. However, the most limitation of this medical aid is that G551D mutation is there in just a pair of 2.3% patients [41]. It is not found to be effective within the commonest F508del (class II) mutation owing to reduced accessibility of protein. In addition, the high price of medical aid may additionally be a limiting reason (ICER: £335,000–£1,274,000/ QALYs gained) [42].

3.3.4.3 Lumacaftor

Another CFTR modulator, lumacaftor, has revealed favorable leads in F508del mutation. This is the main common mutation influencing more or less one-third of

CF population in USA and nearly 70% in EU. This mutation affects the warmth steadiness because of misfolding of NBD1 field and limits the CFTR in ER for succeeding degradation. It did not succeed to localize to proper epithelial site and attain regular formation. Exaggerated transfer of protein to cell surface was ascertained in vitro by means of cultured individual bronchial epithelium [43]. Still, despite exaggerated transfer of protein to correct position, no rectification of the underlying functional impairment was ascertained. Besides, another in vitro study exposed disparity in negative results [44] that were more strengthened by a trial. No vital improvement was ascertained in FEV1, CFQR scores, and respiratory exacerbation rates [45].

3.3.4.4 Orkambi

The approval of CFTR modulators, Kalydeco™ (ivacaftor) and Orkambi™ (lumacaftor/ivacaftor), marks two mile stones in our pursuit of 'a cure' for people suffering from CF. Firstly, phase II trials were performed for each homozygous and heterozygous F508del patients >12 years old; however, solely homozygous patients confirmed clinically noteworthy results. Two massive phase III trials, TRAFFIC and TRANSPORT, were conducted with the mix medical aid (600 + 250 and 400 + 250 mg versus placebo) in patients ≥12 years with primary end as FEV1 improvement at 24 weeks. Patients finishing the study were progressed to 48 weeks PROGRESS trial. The isolated plus pooled outcomes showed a noteworthy improvement in parameters as well as FEV1, reduction of exacerbations, decline in hospitalizations, and rise in BMI and CFQR scores. The undesirable effects were comparable to placebo cluster except one case of death throughout the extension period [46, 47]. In addition, a phase I clinical trial study in homozygous kids ≤12 years showed promising results; however, more advanced phase studies are required [47]. However, in comparison to ivacaftor monotherapy in patients including G551D mutation during a separate study, there was considerably less improvement in pneumonic performed with combination medical aid [3]. Orkambi (lumacaftor + ivacaftor) is permitted recently for homozygous F508del patients ≥12 years. Orkambi acts by a two-step technique. Lumacaftor assists in moving the defective protein to its accurate site and ivacaftor rectifies and enhances its activity eventually escalating the conductance of ions and fluid.

3.3.5 Drawbacks of Current Treatment

Although over 2000 variants in the CFTR gene have been identified to date, F508del accounts for most CFTR alleles in patients with CF, there is still a little restriction that embody (a) non-considerable reply in F508del mutation heterozygotes by ivacaftor; (b) got to keep on further daily symptomatic cure; (c) contact with CYP3A inducers and inhibitors; (d) adverse effects together with elevated transaminases, cataract, oropharyngeal pain and URTI; (e) negligible profit in <12 years old; (f) require of upper prescribed amount up to 600 mg (during case of lumacaftor); and (g) common contact of lumacaftor and ivacaftor leading to improved metabolism of ivacaftor and require of a upper prescribed amount blend. Furthermore, on account of the multi domain formation and in order folding of CFTR, no solo "corrector drug" can repair all the misfolding in dissimilar domains, so a mixture of drugs is a necessity. Furthermore, from a clinical trial viewpoint, there are sample size problems, as precise criteria (major and minor endpoints) make choice more complicated before narrowed mutation precise inhabitants deserve exclusive adaptive trial designs [48].

3.3.6 Future Directions in Therapeutics

CF management does not solely need CFTR correction and modification; however, intensive symptomatic treatment targets inflammation, infection, bronchial hydration, and nutrition. Newer medicines targeting these problems are summed up below in short.

3.3.6.1 Inflammation

Andecaliximab, which is a protein to matrix metalloproteinase 9 (MMP9), is undergoing phase IIb and is expected to cut back inflammation and improve lung task. However, the baseline FEV1 needed for this drug is between 40% and 80% limiting its use in terribly severe CF [49]. An additional compound in phase 1 is POL6014 that is synthesized to dam neutrophil elastase operation, finally reducing the tissue damage and lung inflammation. LAU-7b, perhaps a fenretinide, is a component of retinoid compounds associated with vitamin A. Phase 2 study is thus far to start and it is expected to cut back the inflammatory response in CF lungs. CTX-4430 decreases the making of leukotriene B4, an inflammatory intermediary enhances in CF. It is currently undergoing a phase 2 trial [50]. Additional anti-inflammatory compounds within clinical progress pipeline are α-1 anti-trypsin, CTX-4430, enzyme substance AZD9668, JBT-101 (phase 2) for reducing inflammation.

3.3.6.2 Hydration and Mucus Secretion Clearance

AZD5634 is undergoing section 1b study. It is anticipated to dam the metal channel in CF airway, therefore rehydrating and tapering the mucus secretion within the lungs, creating it easier to clear. SPX-101 is one more compound designed to dam sodium channel operation within the lungs, presently undergoing phase 2 study. OrPro (ORP-100) may be a changed variety of thioredoxin, probably to lessen mucus thickness within the lungs and recover clearance from the CF airway. OligoG (Alginate Oligosaccharide) has revealed to decline mucus viscosity in CF airway. It is presently being tested in phase IIb in Europe and UK. It is often used either as a dry powder or fluid meant for nebulization [51].

Additional agents for rehydration of airway secretions comprise of *bronchitol* presently in phase 3 in USA and by now permitted in UK, Australia, and Russia (for patients >18 years); VX-371 (P1037) presently in phase 2 for obstructing sodium channel and delaying the length of hypertonic saline alone in subjects with cystic fibrosis [52]; GSK2225745 acting by calming ENaC during RNA intervention is ongoing to get in touch with the patients.

3.3.6.3 Nutrition

Liprotamase (Anthera AN-EPI 3332), perhaps pancreatic enzyme substitution for CF-associated pancreatic insufficiency, is undergoing phase 3 study [53].

AquADEKs-2 experience phase 2 may be a balanced blend of fat-soluble vitamins and numerous antioxidants as well as beta-carotene, mixed tocopherols, coenzyme Q10, mixed carotenoids, and minerals like zinc and selenium. Oral glutathione is being tried in phase 2 because this antioxidant is mainly for usual lung GIT operation.CF patients have delineated inferior glutathione levels and oral glutathione is probable to enhance growth and reduce gut inflammation [54]. Additional agents like protein *burlulipase* for pancreatic deficiency, *lubiprostone* for constipation and *roscovitine* for pulmonary contamination are presently being assessed at numerous centers.

3.4 Perspective

Gene engineering skills and novel molecular objective could also be explored further examination of this region led to the identification of the gene itself and the prediction of the amino acid sequence of the encoded protein, which was termed the CFTR (cystic fibrosis transmembrane conductance regulator). Assistance of current biology moves toward like DNA engineering, systems biology, metabolomics, ailment modeling, and intracellular protein kinetics could facilitate to unknot novel pathways and networks associated with cystic fibrosis and ultimately novel therapeutic targets. Also, the focus ought not to be reduced on new treatment techniques, new medicine for symptomatic progression and difficulty avoidance.

References

1. Meyerholz DK, Stoltz DA, Namati E, Ramachandran S, Pezzulo AA, Smith AR, Rector MV, Suter MJ, Kao S, McLennan G, Tearney GJ, Zabner J, McCray PB Jr, Welsh MJ (2010) Loss of cystic fibrosis transmembrane conductance regulator function produces abnormalities in tracheal development in neonatal pigs and young children. Am J Respir Crit Care Med 182 (10):1251–1261
2. Stoltz DA, Meyerholz DK, Pezzulo AA, Ramachandran S, Rogan MP, Davis GJ, Hanfland RA, Wohlford-Lenane C, Dohrn CL, Bartlett JA, Nelson GA IV, Chang EH, Taft PJ, Ludwig PS, Estin M, Hornick EE, Launspach JL, Samuel M, Rokhlina T, Karp PH, Ostedgaard LS, Uc A, Starner TD, Horswill AR, Brogden KA, Prather RS, Richter SS, Shilyansky J, McCray PB Jr, Zabner J, Welsh MJ (2010) Cystic fibrosis pigs develop lung disease and exhibit defective bacterial eradication at birth. Sci Transl Med 2(29):29ra31
3. Accurso FJ, Rowe SM, Clancy JP, Boyle MP, Dunitz JM, Durie PR, Sagel SD, Hornick DB, Konstan MW, Donaldson SH, Moss RB, Pilewski JM, Rubenstein RC, Uluer AZ, Aitken ML, Freedman SD, Rose LM, Mayer-Hamblett N, Dong Q, Zha J, Stone AJ, Olson ER, Ordoñez CL,

Campbell PW, Ashlock MA, Ramsey BW (2010) Effect of VX-770 in persons with cystic fibrosis and the G551D-CFTR mutation. N Engl J Med 363(21):1991–2003
4. Muhlebach MS, Stewart PW, Leigh MW, Noah TL (1999) Quantitation of inflammatory responses to bacteria in young cystic fibrosis and control patients. Am J Respir Crit Care Med 160(1):186–191
5. Sly PD (2013) Risk factors for bronchiectasis in children with cystic fibrosis. N Engl J Med 368 (21):1963–1970
6. Tiringer K, Treis A, Fucik P, Gona M, Gruber S, Renner S, Dehlink E, Nachbaur E, Horak F, Jaksch P, Döring G, Crameri R, Jung A, Rochat MK, Hörmann M, Spittler A, Klepetko W, Akdis CA, Szépfalusi Z, Frischer T, Eiwegger T (2013) A Th17-and Th2-skewed cytokine profile in cystic fibrosis lungs represents a potential risk factor for Pseudomonas aeruginosa infection. Am J Respir Crit Care Med 187(6):621–629
7. Lloyd-Still JD (1994) Crohn's disease and cystic fibrosis. Dig Dis Sci 39(4):880–885
8. Kumar S, Tana A, Shankar A (2014) Cystic fibrosis-what are the prospects for a cure? Eur J Intern Med 25(9):803–807
9. WHO (2018) Genes human disease-cystic fibrosis. WHO, Geneva, Switzerland
10. Riordan JR, Rommens JM, Kerem B, Alon N, Rozmahel R, Grzelczak Z, Zielenski J, Lok S, Plavsic N, Chou JL (1989) Identification of the cystic fibrosis gene: cloning and characterization of complementary DNA. Science 245(4922):1066–1073
11. Pezzulo AA, Tang XX, Hoegger MJ, Abou Alaiwa MH, Ramachandran S, Moninger TO, Karp PH, Wohlford-Lenane CL, Haagsman HP, van Eijk M, Bánfi B, Horswill AR, Stoltz DA, McCray PB Jr, Welsh MJ, Zabner J (2012) Reduced airway surface pH impairs bacterial killing in the porcine cystic fibrosis lung. Nature 487(7405):109
12. Vonberg RP, Gastmeier P (2005) Isolation of infectious cystic fibrosis patients: results of a systematic review. Infect Cont Hosp Epidemiol 26(4):401–409
13. Liou TG, Adler FR, Fitzsimmons SC, Cahill BC, Hibbs JR, Marshall BC (2001) Predictive 5-year survivorship model of cystic fibrosis. Am J Epidemiol 153(4):345–352
14. Hart N, Polkey MI, Clément A, Boulé M, Moxham J, Lofaso F, Fauroux B (2002) Changes in pulmonary mechanics with increasing disease severity in children and young adults with cystic fibrosis. Am J Respir Crit Care Med 166(1):61–66
15. Saadane A, Soltys J, Berger M (2005) Role of IL-10 deficiency in excessive nuclear factor-κB activation and lung inflammation in cystic fibrosis transmembrane conductance regulator knockout mice. J Allergy Clin Immunol 115(2):405–411
16. Antonelli M, Midulla F, Tancredi G, Salvatori FM, Bonci E, Cimino G, Flaishman I (2002) Bronchial artery embolization for the management of nonmassive hemoptysis in cystic fibrosis. Chest 121(3):796–801
17. Orenstein DM, Winnie GB, Altman H (2002) Cystic fibrosis: a 2002 update. J Pediatr 140 (2):156–164
18. Marchand E et al (2001) Frequency of cystic fibrosis transmembrane conductance regulator gene mutations and 5T allele in patients with allergic bronchopulmonary aspergillosis. Chest 119(3):762–767
19. Venarske DL, de Shazo RD (2002) Sinobronchial allergic mycosis: the SAM syndrome. Chest 121(5):1670–1676
20. Elphick HE, Southern KW (2016) Antifungal therapies for allergic bronchopulmonary aspergillosis in people with cystic fibrosis. Cochrane Database Syst Rev (11):CD002204
21. Mange EJ, Mange AP (1999) Basic human genetics. Sinauer Associates, Sunderland, MA
22. Stites SW, Plautz MW, Bailey K, O'Brien-Ladner AR, Wesselius LJ (1999) Increased concentrations of iron and isoferritins in the lower respiratory tract of patients with stable cystic fibrosis. Am J Respir Crit Care Med 160(3):796–801
23. Taussig L (1999) Pediatric respiratory medicine. Mosby, St Louis, MO
24. Brunzell C, Schwarzenberg SJ (2002) Cystic fibrosis-related diabetes and abnormal glucose tolerance: overview and medical nutrition therapy. Diabet Spect 15(2):124–127

25. Moran A, Hardin D, Rodman D, Allen HF, Beall RJ, Borowitz D, Brunzell C, Campbell PW III, Chesrown SE, Duchow C, Fink RJ, Fitzsimmons SC, Hamilton N, Hirsch I, Howenstine MS, Klein DJ, Madhun Z, Pencharz PB, Quittner AL, Robbins MK, Schindler T, Schissel K, Schwarzenberg SJ, Stallings VA, Zipf WB (1999) Diagnosis, screening and management of cystic fibrosis related diabetes mellitus: a consensus conference report. Diabetes Res Clin Pract 45(1):61–73
26. Moss RB (2002) Long-term benefits of inhaled tobramycin in adolescent patients with cystic fibrosis. Chest 121(1):55–63
27. Konstan MW, Flume PA, Kappler M, Chiron R, Higgins M, Brockhaus F, Zhang J, Angyalosi G, He E, Geller DE (2011) Safety, efficacy and convenience of tobramycin inhalation powder in cystic fibrosis patients: the EAGER trial. J Cyst Fibros 10(1):54–61
28. Flume PA, O'Sullivan BP, Robinson KA, Goss CH, Mogayzel PJ Jr, Willey-Courand DB, Bujan J, Finder J, Lester M, Quittell L, Rosenblatt R, Vender RL, Hazle L, Sabadosa K, Marshall B, Cystic Fibrosis Foundation, Pulmonary Therapies Committee (2007) Cystic fibrosis pulmonary guidelines: chronic medications for maintenance of lung health. Am J Respir Crit Care Med 176(10):957–969
29. Salvatore D, D'Andria M (2002) Effects of salmeterol on arterial oxyhemoglobin saturations in patients with cystic fibrosis. Pediatr Pulmonol 34(1):11–15
30. Robinson M, Regnis JA, Bailey DL, King M, Bautovich GJ, Bye PT (1996) Effect of hypertonic saline, amiloride, and cough on mucociliary clearance in patients with cystic fibrosis. Am J Respir Crit Care Med 153(5):1503–1509
31. Quan JM, Tiddens HA, Sy JP, McKenzie SG, Montgomery MD, Robinson PJ, Wohl ME, Konstan MW, Pulmozyme Early Intervention Trial Study Group (2001) A two-year randomized, placebo-controlled trial of dornase alfa in young patients with cystic fibrosis with mild lung function abnormalities. J Pediatr 139(6):813–820
32. McIlwaine MP, Alarie N, Davidson GF, Lands LC, Ratjen F, Milner R, Owen B, Agnew JL (2013) Long-term multicentre randomised controlled study of high frequency chest wall oscillation versus positive expiratory pressure mask in cystic fibrosis. Thorax 68(8):746–751
33. Colombo C, Ellemunter H, Houwen R, Munck A, Taylor C, Wilschanski M, ECFS (2011) Guidelines for the diagnosis and management of distal intestinal obstruction syndrome in cystic fibrosis patients. J Cyst Fibros 10:S24–S28
34. Stern RC, Eisenberg JD, Wagener JS, Ahrens R, Rock M, do Pico G, Orenstein DM (2000) A comparison of the efficacy and tolerance of pancrelipase and placebo in the treatment of steatorrhea in cystic fibrosis patients with clinical exocrine pancreatic insufficiency. Am J Gastroenterol 95(8):1932
35. Borowitz D, Borowitz D, Robinson KA, Rosenfeld M, Davis SD, Sabadosa KA, Spear SL, Michel SH, Parad RB, White TB, Farrell PM, Marshall BC, Accurso FJ (2009) Cystic Fibrosis Foundation evidence-based guidelines for management of infants with cystic fibrosis. J Pediatr 155(6):S73–S93
36. Vertex Pharmaceuticals Inc (2012) Kalydeco™ (ivacaftor). Product Information. Cambridge
37. Ramsey BW (2011) A CFTR potentiator in patients with cystic fibrosis and the G551D mutation. N Engl J Med 365(18):1663–1672
38. Davies JC (2013) Efficacy and safety of ivacaftor in patients aged 6 to 11 years with cystic fibrosis with a G551D mutation. Am J Respir Crit Care Med 187(11):1219–1225
39. Davies JC, Cunningham S, Harris WT, Lapey A, Regelmann WE, Sawicki GS, Southern KW, Robertson S, Green Y, Cooke J, Rosenfeld M, KIWI Study Group (2016) Safety, pharmacokinetics, and pharmacodynamics of ivacaftor in patients aged 2-5 years with cystic fibrosis and a CFTR gating mutation (KIWI): an open-label, single-arm study. Lancet Respir Med 4(2):107–115
40. Rowe SM, Heltshe SL, Gonska T, Donaldson SH, Borowitz D, Gelfond D, Sagel SD, Khan U, Mayer-Hamblett N, Van Dalfsen JM, Joseloff E, Ramsey BW, GOAL Investigators of the Cystic Fibrosis Foundation Therapeutics Development Network (2014) Clinical mechanism of

the cystic fibrosis transmembrane conductance regulator potentiator ivacaftor in G551D-mediated cystic fibrosis. Am J Respir Crit Care Med 190(2):175–184
41. (2016) http://www.who.int/genomics/publications/en/HGN_WB_04.02_report.pdf
42. Whiting P, Burgers L, Westwood M, Ryder S, Hoogendoorn M, Armstrong N, Allen A, Severens H, Kleijnen J (2014) Ivacaftor for the treatment of patients with cystic fibrosis and the G551D mutation: a systematic review and cost-effectiveness analysis. Health Technol Assess 18(18):1–106
43. Van Goor F, Hadida S, Grootenhuis PD, Burton B, Stack JH, Straley KS, Decker CJ, Miller M, McCartney J, Olson ER, Wine JJ, Frizzell RA, Ashlock M, Negulescu PA (2011) Correction of the F508del-CFTR protein processing defect in vitro by the investigational drug VX-809. Proc Natl Acad Sci 108(46):18843–18848
44. Kopeikin Z, Yuksek Z, Yang HY, Bompadre SG (2014) Combined effects of VX-770 and VX-809 on several functional abnormalities of F508del-CFTR channels. J Cyst Fibros 13 (5):508–514
45. Clancy J, Rowe SM, Accurso FJ, Aitken ML, Amin RS, Ashlock MA, Ballmann M, Boyle MP, Bronsveld I, Campbell PW, De Boeck K, Donaldson SH, Dorkin HL, Dunitz JM, Durie PR, Jain M, Leonard A, McCoy KS, Moss RB, Pilewski JM, Rosenbluth DB, Rubenstein RC, Schechter MS, Botfield M, Ordoñez CL, Spencer-Green GT, Vernillet L, Wisseh S, Yen K, Konstan MW (2012) Results of a phase IIa study of VX-809, an investigational CFTR corrector compound, in subjects with cystic fibrosis homozygous for the F508del-CFTR mutation. Thorax 67(1):12–18
46. Ramsey B, Elborn S (2014) Effect of lumacaftor in combination with ivacaftor in patients with cystic fibrosis who are homozygous for F508del-CFTR: pooled results from the phase 3 TRAFFIC and TRANSPORT studies. In: The 28th Annual North American Conference of the Cystic Fibrosis Foundation, Atlanta, GA
47. Wainwright CE (2015) Lumacaftor–ivacaftor in patients with cystic fibrosis homozygous for Phe508del CFTR. N Engl J Med 373(3):220–231
48. Rafeeq MM, Murad HAS (2017) Cystic fibrosis: current therapeutic targets and future approaches. J Transl Med 15(1):84
49. Gilead Sciences (2018) A phase 2b, dose-ranging study of the effect of GS-5745 on FEV1 in adult subjects with cystic fibrosis
50. Steven Rowe M, Stuart Elborn MD (2019) A phase 2, multicenter, randomized, double-blind, placebo-controlled, parallel-group study to evaluate the efficacy, safety, and tolerability of CTX-4430 administered orally once-daily for 48 weeks in adult patients with cystic fibrosis
51. Tacjana Pressler PM (2017) A double-blind, randomized, placebo-controlled cross over study of inhaled alginate oligosaccharide (OligoG) administered for 28 days in subjects with cystic fibrosis
52. Vertex Pharmaceuticals Inc (2017) A phase 2a, randomized, double-blind, placebo-controlled, incomplete block, crossover study to evaluate the safety and efficacy of VX-371 in subjects aged 12 years or older with cystic fibrosis, homozygous for the F508del-CFTR mutation, and being treated with Orkambi
53. Anthera Pharmaceuticals (2018) A phase 3, open-label study evaluating the efficacy and safety of liprotamase in subjects with cystic fibrosis-related exocrine pancreatic insufficiency
54. Sarah J, Schwarzenberg M, Sarah J Schwarzenberg MD (2018) A multi center placebo controlled double blind randomized study evaluating the role of oral glutathione on growth parameters in children with cystic fibrosis

Chronic Pneumonia

4

Shravan Kumar Paswan, Vishal Kumar Vishwakarma,
Chetan Rastogi, Pritt Verma, Ch. V. Rao, and Sajal Srivastava

Abstract

Chronic eosinophilic pneumonia (CEP) is associated with eosinophilic lung ailment specifically/usually diagnosed by a triad of clinical warning signs together with pulmonary warning signs, eosinophilia, as well as distinguishing radiographic defects. It needs a high indicator of doubt given that it is overlain with other eosinophilic situations and be deficient in a diagnostic assay. The diagnosis is made after careful consideration of other secondary causes of eosinophilia, such as infectious, drugs, or toxic etiologies. CEP generally responds rapidly to treatment, which primarily consists of corticosteroid therapy, but relapses are common. New remedies are being investigated which are documented in new studies regarding the pathophysiology of eosinophilic illness progression. Close follow-up is important given the difficulty in weaning patients from glucocorticoids with many patients developing sequelae of chronic glucocorticoid therapy. Hence, searching for various treatments is being prioritized by the scientific community.

Keywords

Chronic eosinophilic pneumonia (CEP) · Common variable immunological disorder (CVID) · Mepolizumab · Omalizumab · BAL

S. K. Paswan (✉) · P. Verma · C. V. Rao
Pharmacology Division, CSIR-National Botanical Research Institute, Lucknow, Uttar Pradesh, India
e-mail: paswanshravan@gmail.com

V. K. Vishwakarma
Department of Pharmacology, All India Institute of Medical Sciences (AIIMS), New Delhi, India

C. Rastogi
King George Medical University, Lucknow, Uttar Pradesh, India

S. Srivastava
Amity Institute of Pharmacy, Amity University Uttar Pradesh, Lucknow, Uttar Pradesh, India

S. Rayees et al. (eds.), *Chronic Lung Diseases*,
https://doi.org/10.1007/978-981-15-3734-9_4

4.1 Introduction

4.1.1 About the Disease

Eosinophilic lung diseases are a group of diffuse parenchymal lung diseases characterized by the prominent infiltration of the lung interstitial and alveolar spaces by polymorphonuclear eosinophils, with conservation of the lung architecture. As a corollary, a common denominator of eosinophilic lung diseases is represented by a dramatic response to systemic corticosteroid therapy and healing without any sequelae in most cases, despite frequent impressive impairment of lung function at presentation [1]. CEP was first recognized as a unique pulmonary entity in 1969, characterized by Carrington et al., when a series of female patients were described as presenting with symptoms of dyspnea, fever, and weight loss who demonstrated pulmonary opacities on chest X-ray and had noted eosinophilic infiltration on lung biopsy specimens. The condition is thought to be idiopathic, with no known infectious or toxic etiology identified. CEP is a clinical diagnosis and has a presentation that is typically described as a triad of the following: pulmonary symptoms, abnormal chest imaging, and abnormal elevation of eosinophils in either serum or pulmonary tissue [2].

4.1.2 Epidemiology

Representing <3% of cases of varied interstitial diseases, CEP may be a rare illness. It is, however, the foremost common of the eosinophilic pneumonias in nontropical areas wherever incidence of parasitic infections is low. Most patients are nonsmokers, and it is thought that <10% diagnosed are smokers. This contrasts with acute leucocyte respiratory illness within which a smoking history is a far lot in common [3]. It is a significant reason behind death among all age groups, leading to 1.4 million deaths in 2010 (7% of the world's yearly total) and was the fourth leading reason behind death within the world in 2016, leading to 3 million deaths worldwide [4, 5].

4.1.3 Causes/Symptoms

A cluster of disorders is classified by etiology, together with secondary causes like infectious, malignant, allergic, drug, and deadly etiologies. Primary eosinophilic lung diseases can be further classified by isolated pneumonic involvement vs. general involvement, and two major isolated pneumonic white blood cell respiratory organ diseases embody acute eosinophilic pneumonia (AEP) and CEP, though these are commonly less abundant [2].

4.2 Pathophysiology of Pneumonia

4.2.1 Cell Types Involved

There is a complex balance amid the organisms residing within the lower tract and also the native and general defense mechanisms (both innate and acquired) that once disturbed give rise to inflammation of the respiratory organ parenchyma, i.e., pneumonia. Common defense mechanisms that are compromised within the pathologic process of respiratory illness include:

- Systemic defense mechanisms like body substance and complement-mediated immunity that is compromised in diseases like common variable immunological disorder (CVID), X-linked immunodeficiency (inherited), and purposeful as plenia (acquired). Impaired cell-mediated immunity predisposes people to infection by living organisms like viruses and organisms of low virulence like pneumonia (PJP), plant causes, among others.
- The mucociliary clearance that is usually impaired in cigarette smokers, post-viral state, Kartergerner syndrome, and different connected conditions.
- Impaired cough reflex seen in comatose patients, a sure indication of substance abuse.
- Accumulation of secretions as seen in mucoviscidosis or in cartilaginous tube obstruction.

The resident macrophages serve to safeguard the respiratory organ from foreign pathogens. Ironically, the inflammatory reaction triggered by these terrible macrophages is what is chargeable for the histopathological and clinical findings seen in respiratory illness. The macrophages engulf these pathogens and trigger signal molecules or cytokines like TNF-α, IL-8, and IL-1 that recruit inflammatory cells like neutrophils to the positioning of infection. They conjointly serve to gift these antigens to the T cells that trigger each cellular and body substance defense mechanisms and activate the targeted antibodies against these organisms. This, in turn, causes inflammation of the respiratory organ parenchyma and makes the liner capillaries leaky, resulting in oxidative congestion and underlines the pathologic process of respiratory illness [6].

4.2.2 Biology of the Disease

Eosinophils are multifunctional leukocytes involved in innate and reconciling immunity. They mature within the bone marrow beneath stimulation from cytokines. Particularly, they are influenced by IL-5, IL-3, granulocyte-macrophage colony-stimulating tissue, and transcription factors including delta-dbl-GATA-1, before disseminating into the blood and after into tissues. Eosinophils have intra-cytoplasmic granules containing proteins, toxins, and chemokines, and pro-inflammatory degranulation of eosinophils releases these venomous substances

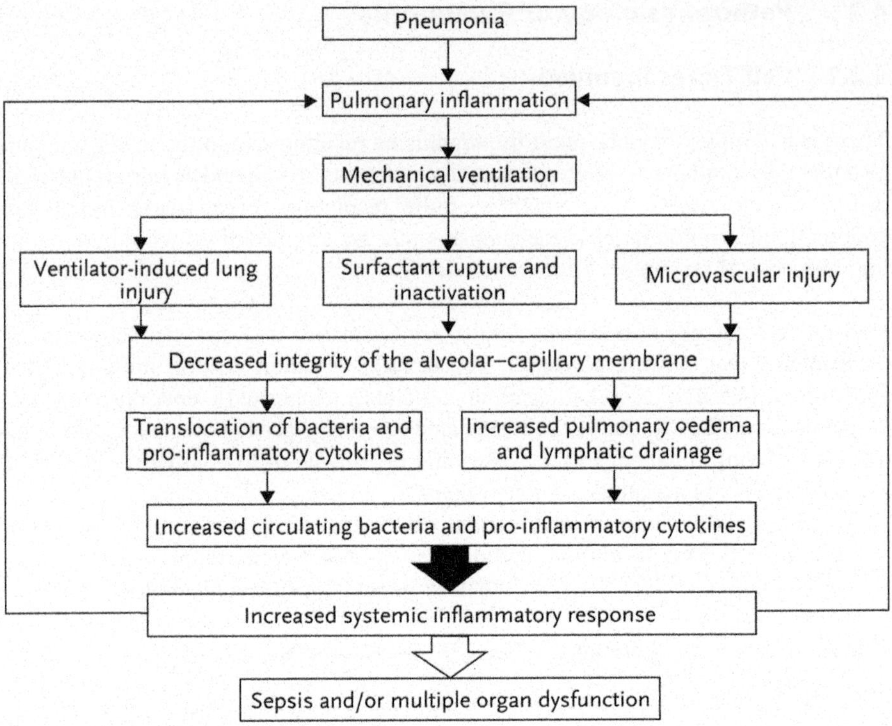

Fig. 4.1 Biology of the disease

into the tissues, which contributes to the pathophysiology of WBC disorders (Fig. 4.1). Eosinophils move with multiple cellular pathways, as well as T helper lymphocytes, mast cells and basophils, macrophages, and multiple cells. However, the white corpuscle play an important role in respiratory organ and it principally directed by IL-5 and also the eotaxin taxonomic category of chemokines [7]. Additionally, recent study suggests that IL-25 might uphold chronic WBC inflammation of the respiratory organ [8]. Histopathological lesions are associated with the toxicity of small piece discharge of eosinophils and are mostly reversible with treatment, though tissue harm and reworking will be seen [7]. Osteopontin levels are found to be elevated in bronchoalveolar lavage (BAL) fluid of patients with WBC respiratory illness as well as drug-induced eosinophilic pneumonia. They will play a role in WBC inflammation [1].

4.2.3 Transcriptional Regulation

The interface between the external environment (including microbes therein) and the internal environment (including leukocytes and other immune cells) is the respiratory epithelium, and immunity roles of this interface were the subject of extensive study. We learned that an essential action of the cytokine IL-17, already well recognized for driving sterilizing immunity against extracellular bacteria and fungi, is to activate the lung's epithelial lining. IL-17 signals to cells via the IL-17RA receptor, and it has become apparent that humans with mutations in IL-17RA show greater susceptibilities to bacterial pneumonia. Although IL-17 receptors are expressed by many different cell types, the mutation of IL-17RA in lung epithelial cells selectively (in mice with CC10-Cre transgenes and floxed ***Il17ra***) was demonstrated to be sufficient to increase bacterial burdens during *Klebsiella pneumoniae* pneumonia in mice. A protective action observed was the induction of CXCL5 by epithelial cells, advancing prior studies that suggested this was an epithelial-specific product during pneumonia that elicits neutrophil recruitment. Transcriptional profiling experiments in mice with pneumococcal pneumonia have now revealed that CXCL5 is only one of many hundreds of genes that are induced preferentially in epithelial cells during infection, dozens of which are secreted products like CXCL5 that can mediate immune cell cross-talk. Another epithelial-specific product was identified as a neutrophil activator, secreted and transmembrane 1 (Sectm1), which stimulates recruited neutrophils to make more of the neutrophil-attracting chemokine, CXCL2, thereby amplifying the positive feedback of inflammation within the infected lung. Harnessing the power of epithelial innate immunity, pharmacologically triggering these cells is being pursued as a means to provide protection against diverse respiratory infections, and it now appears that this can be effective even in mice modeling leukemia patients, despite profound immune dysregulation due to both leukemia and leukemia treatment.

4.3 Current Treatment

The mainstay of treatment relies on oral corticosteroid (OCS) therapy; with a goal of causing remission further as reducing the chance of reversion [9]. Response to OCS is sometimes dramatic and fast, with each clinical improvement and backbone of infiltrates on imaging. It is worth noting that response generally happens within many days, and if fast clinical improvement is not seen, various diagnoses ought to be reconsidered [10]. Low-dose inhaled corticosteroids (ICS) were used formerly to help with tapering and discontinuing OCS. ICS have thus been planned as monotherapy, thanks to the suspected deposition of ICS in alveoli to stop the event of the aspect effects from long-run usage of OCS. However, a study performed by Minakuchi et al. suggests that ICS might not be a good monotherapy. While not treatment, spontaneous resolution happens in $<10\%$ of patients with CEP, and is a near threat of succession to fibrosis [11].

There are no firm doses or period tips. The general goal is to keep up continued clinical improvement on very cheap attainable dose of OCS so as to avoid relapse but conjointly minimize steroid-related facet effects. Initial treatment is usually with oral prednisone at 0.5–0.6 mg/kg/day with the dose narrowing down by a common fraction on confirmation of each clinical and radiologic resolution [12]. A review of this literature relating to treatment by Suzuki et al. suggests that a beginning dose of prednisolone of around 30 mg would be adequate [10]. Treatment periods are variable from several months to 12 months, depending on the clinical response. Relapses are common, occurring in over half the patients [9]. Despite this typically accepted observe, only one study so far has prospectively evaluated the optimum treatment plan with relevance to reversion rate, in an exceedingly irregular parallel-group study. In this trial, the study cluster received the OCS treatment at a daily dose of 0.5 mg/kg/day over a shorter 3-month period compared to an equivalent dose in an exceedingly longer 6-month period. Within the 3-month cluster, the prednisolone was tapered by 20% each 2 weeks to nil by 3 months, whereas within the 6-month cluster, the prednisolone was tapered off slower over 6 months. They were determined for 2 years on completion of treatment. The relapse rates were similar between the teams (52.1% vs. 61.9%, $P = 0.56$), suggesting that a shorter treatment amount is also acceptable, with revised observation [13].

4.3.1 Drawbacks of the Current Treatment

Although the extensive tenure prognosis of the illness is highly sensitive to systemic corticosteroids, but frequently relapses if the dose is tapered or treatment discontinued. Partly patients are noted to suffer reversion, with some failure numerous times. Commencement of OCS medical therapy in relapsed cases is uniformly effective. Predictors of relapse have not been strictly evaluated; however smoking underlying bronchial asthma are double risk factors [10, 14]. These patients might need chronic steroid maintenance medical care, and efforts to mitigate aspect effects are necessary [10]. This additionally leads to efforts toward finding probable steroid-reducing therapies.

4.3.2 Future Directions in Therapeutics

Most of other therapies are delineated just in case of reports with no strong proof supporting their use in CEP. Omalizumab, an antibody against IgE, was utilized in a patient with CEP on the second reversion in 2 years. This patient had an elevated IgE and had been given omalizumab injections. The patient was deemed to be sickness-free after 15 months of medical aid [15]. During a succeeding case report, Domingo et al. delineated a fortunate use of omalizumab in a patient with CEP with distinguished asthmatic options and mud mite allergen. They were ready to taper the dose of omalizumab by 500 mg each for 6 months [16]. Clinicians ought to be tuned in to the chance of exposure to eosinophilic granulomatosis with polyangiitis (EGPA) in these patients [15].

There are many alternative potential targets for CEP, most ordinarily against IL-5. Amplified levels of IL-5 with associated discharge of cytotoxic granular proteins from eosinophils are a decisive mechanism into the pathophysiology of CEP [17].

Mepolizumab and reslizumab stop binding of circulating IL-5 to eosinophils. Benralizumab neutralizes IL-5 and operates by binding the alpha fractional subunit of the IL-5 receptor and is additionally ready to induce programmed cell death of target cells via antibody-dependent cell-mediated toxicity [18, 19]. During a massive multicenter randomized controlled trial involving 621 patients, mepolizumab reduced the speed of asthma attack exacerbations in rigorous eosinophilic asthma [20]. It has conjointly been demonstrated to cut back the frequency of asthma attack exacerbations and is identified to be helpful as a possible steroid-sparing agent in hyper eosinophilic syndromes [21, 22]. Although anti-IL5 therapies are verified as efficacious in eosinophilic asthma attack, there is restricted knowledge on the employment of those therapies in CEP.

A recent report delineated a patient with CEP who had undergone glucocorticoid medical aid, however failing steroid taper and experienced noteworthy steroid-induced side effects together with weight gain, Cushingoid options, and muscle wasting. Eighteen months subsequent to preliminary appearance, mepolizumab was started at a dose of 100 mg each for 4 weeks. Once this medical aid commenced, her peripheral blood symptoms weakened, and her symptoms disappeared whereas tapering of glucocorticoids was found. However, she developed a gentle hypersensitivity reaction subsequent to 6 months of medical aid. Therefore, reslizumab at a dose of 3 mg/kg was initiated each for 4 weeks. Following 2 further months, she was ready for discontinuing her glucocorticoids [23]. Mepolizumab had conjointly been used effectively in another patient with CEP and a 20-year history of asthma attack throughout his second reversion at 100 mg each month [24]. However, the period of medical aid with mepolizumab in such patients remains unclear.

Other potential targets for treatment of CEP embrace IL-25, IL-33, IL-4, and IL-13. IL-25 and IL-33 are first and foremost made by airway epithelial cells that induce the assembly of Th2-type cytokines together with IL-5 and IL-13 on eosinophils. Katoh et al. examined the BAL fluid in 20 with AEP, 22 patients with CEP, 20 with idiopathic pulmonary fibrosis (IPF), and 20 with sarcoidosis. Patients with acute and chronic eosinophilic asthma attacks had higher IL-5 and eosinophil levels compared to patients with IPF and sarcoidosis. Curiously, IL-25 levels were elevated in patients with CEP, however not AEP. IL-33 levels were not considerably totally different in eosinophilic pneumonia when compared to sarcoidosis and IPF [8]. The results of this study indicate that IL-25 could also be a possible therapeutic target for CEP. Currently, antibodies to Il-25 do not seem to be commercially offered.

Dupilumab may be a human anti-IL-4 receptor α-monoclonal protein that targets each IL-4 and IL-13 communication and thus TH2-type inflammation. Fidel Castro Ruz et al. at random appointed 1902 patients to varied doses of dupilumab vs. placebo and confirmed reduced frequency of asthma attack exacerbation and improvement in forced expiratory volume in 1 s. In addition, within the Liberty asthma attack Venture trial, add-on dupilumab was ready to considerably cut back the utilization of oral glucocorticoids in patients with severe asthma attack [25]. Dupilumab can also hold promise in designated relapsing cases of CEP; however it has not been utilized in these cases at this point.

4.3.3 Perspective

The short-run viewpoint for patients with CEP is mostly favorable, given the outstanding and timely clinical improvement with corticosteroids. Around half the patients at first diagnosed with CEP have clinical improvement, while there is no relapse or requirement for repeat treatment [26].

Among the remaining half of patients with relapse, repeat OCS dosing or perhaps maintenance of low-dose OCS for long is also needed [26]. In these patients, there is risk of development of steroid-related adverse effects, together with hyperglycemia, diabetes mellitus, osteoporosis, psychosis, and infectious complications like pneumonic non-tuberculoses mycobacterium [10, 14].

In terms of pneumonic status, the bulk of patients with CEP have restriction or obstruction noted on spirometry [15]. Among those with abnormal pneumonic function tests, a majority of patients improve with treatment; however, as many as 37–50% of the patients might have persistent defects after treatment [10, 27].

In summary, given the antecedently mentioned dramatic and fast response in an exceedingly giant share of patients, those who are diagnosed and treated in an exceedingly timely manner might have a good clinical response. Conversely, given the incidence of relapse and also the potential for long-standing steroid-induced side effects or fibrotic changes, more investigations of steroid-sparing therapies like anti-IL5 antibodies are required.

4.4 Toxicokinetics

The most common cause of typical bacterial pneumonia worldwide is *Pneumococcus*. The polysaccharide capsule of *Streptococcus pneumoniae* inhibits the complement binding to the cell surface and hence inhibits phagocytosis. Virulent pneumococcal proteins such as IgA1 protease, neuraminidase, pneumolysin, autolysin, and the surface protein A further help the organism to counteract the host immune response and allow it to cause infection in humans.

Genetic mutations causing an active efflux of drug and eventually resistance have led to an increase in drug-resistant *Streptococcus pneumoniae* (DRSP) over the last few years.

Alteration in penicillin-binding proteins has increased the penicillin resistance and an increased rate of penicillin-resistant *S. pneumoniae*. Penicillin resistance occurs due to failure to bind to the microbe cell wall [28, 29].

4.5 Histopathology

Pathologically, lobar pneumonia is the acute exudative inflammation of a lung lobe. It has the following four advanced stages if left untreated:

1. *Congestion*: In this stage, pulmonary parenchyma is not fully consolidated, and microscopically, the alveoli have serous exudates, pathogens, few neutrophils, and macrophages.
2. *Red Hepatization*: Here, the lobe is now consolidated, firm, and liver-like. Microscopically, there is an addition of fibrin along with serous exudate, pathogens, neutrophils, and macrophages. The capillaries are congested, and the alveolar walls are thickened.
3. *Gray Hepatization*: The lobe is still liver-like in consistency but gray in color due to suppurative and exudative filled alveoli.
4. *Resolution*: After a week, it starts resolving as lymphatic drainage or a productive cough clears the exudates [30].

4.6 History and Physical

The history findings of bacterial pneumonia may vary from indolent to fulminant. Clinical manifestation includes both constitutional findings and findings due to damage to the lung and related tissue. The following are major history findings:

- Fever with tachycardia and/or chills and sweats.
- The cough may be either non-productive or productive with mucoid, purulent, or blood-tinged sputum.
- Pleuritic chest pain, if the pleura is involved.
- Shortness of breath with normal daily routine work.
- Other symptoms include fatigue, headache, myalgia, and arthralgia.

Physical findings also vary from patient to patient and mainly depend on the severity of lung consolidation and existence or nonexistence of pleural effusion. The following are major clinical findings:

- Increased respiratory rate.
- Percussion sounds vary from flat to dull.
- Tactile fremitus.
- Crackles, rales, and bronchial breath sounds are heard on auscultation.

Confusion manifests earlier in older patients. A critically ill patient may present with sepsis or multi-organ failure [31].

4.7 Evaluation

The approach to evaluate and diagnose pneumonia depends on different modalities but primarily it is like a tripod stand which has three legs which are summed up as:

1. *Clinical Evaluation*: It includes taking a careful patient history and performing a thorough physical examination to judge the clinical signs and symptoms mentioned above.
2. *Laboratory Evaluation*: This includes lab values such as complete blood count with differentials, inflammatory biomarkers like ESR and C-reactive protein, blood cultures, sputum analysis, or Gram staining and/or urine antigen testing or polymerase chain reaction for nucleic acid detection of certain bacteria.
3. *Radiological Evaluation*: It includes chest X-ray as an initial imaging test and the finding of pulmonary infiltrates on a plain film is considered as a gold standard for diagnosis when the lab and clinical features are supportive [32, 33].

4.8 Differential Diagnosis

4.8.1 Differential Diagnosis in Children

- Asthma or reactive airway disease
- Bronchiolitis
- Croup
- Respiratory distress syndrome

4.8.2 Differential Diagnosis in Adults

- Acute and chronic bronchitis
- Aspiration of a foreign body
- Asthma
- Atelectasis
- Bronchiectasis
- Bronchiolitis
- Chronic obstructive pulmonary disease
- Fungal
- Lung abscess
- Pneumocystis jiroveci pneumonia
- Respiratory failure
- Viral [34]

4.9 Enhancing Healthcare Team Outcomes

Pneumonia is a common infectious lung disease. It requires interprofessional care and the involvement of more than one subspecialty. This patient-centered approach involving a physician with a team of other health professionals, physiotherapists, respiratory therapists, nurses, pharmacists, and support groups working together for the patient plays an important role in improving the quality of care for pneumonia patients. It not only decreases the hospital admission rates but also positively affects the disease outcome. For healthy patients, the outcomes after treatment are excellent but, in the elderly and those with comorbidities, the outcomes are guarded.

References

1. Cottin V (2016) Eosinophilic lung diseases. Clin Chest Med 37(3):535–556
2. Crowe M, Robinson D, Sagar M, Chen L, Ghamande S (2019) Chronic eosinophilic pneumonia: clinical perspectives. Ther Clin Risk Manag 15:397–403
3. Sevim T, Aksoy E, Akyıl FT, Ağca MÇ, Kongar NA, Özşeker F (2015) Eosinophilic lung disease: accompanied with 12 cases. Turk Thorac J 16(4):172–179
4. Ruuskanen O, Lahti E, Jennings LC, Murdoch DR (2011) Viral pneumonia. Lancet 377 (9773):1264–1275
5. WHO (2018) The top 10 causes of death. www.who.int
6. Mason RJ, Broaddus VC, Martin T, King T, Schraufnagel D, Murray J, Nadel J (2016) Murray and Nadel's textbook of respiratory medicine, 6th edn. Elsevier Saunders, Philadelphia
7. Katoh S, Ikeda M, Matsumoto N, Shimizu H, Abe M, Ohue Y, Mouri K, Kobashi Y, Nakazato M, Oka M (2017) Possible role of IL-25 in eosinophilic lung inflammation in patients with chronic eosinophilic pneumonia. Lung 195(6):707–712
8. Ueno T, Miyazaki E, Ando M, Nureki S, Kumamoto T (2010) Osteopontin levels are elevated in patients with eosinophilic pneumonia. Respirology 15(7):1111–1121
9. Suzuki YT (2018) Suda, long-term management and persistent impairment of pulmonary function in chronic eosinophilic pneumonia: a review of the previous literature. Allergol Int 67(3):334–340
10. Minakuchi M, Niimi A, Matsumoto H, Amitani R, Mishima M (2003) Chronic eosinophilic pneumonia: treatment with inhaled corticosteroids. Respiration 70(4):362–366
11. Marchand E, Cordier JF (2006) Idiopathic chronic eosinophilic pneumonia. Orphanet J Rare Dis 1(1):11
12. Oyama Y, Fujisawa T, Hashimoto D, Enomoto N, Nakamura Y, Inui N, Kuroishi S, Yokomura K, Toyoshima M, Yamada T, Shirai T, Masuda M, Yasuda K, Hayakawa H, Chida K, Suda T (2015) Efficacy of short-term prednisolone treatment in patients with chronic eosinophilic pneumonia. Eur Respir J 45(6):1624–1631
13. Ishiguro T, Takayanagi N, Uozumi R, Tada M, Kagiyama N, Takaku Y, Shimizu Y, Sugita Y, Morita S (2016) The long-term clinical course of chronic eosinophilic pneumonia. Intern Med 55(17):2373–2377
14. Kaya H, Gümüş S, Uçar E, Aydoğan M, Muşabak U, Tozkoparan E, Bilgiç H (2012) Omalizumab as a steroid-sparing agent in chronic eosinophilic pneumonia. Chest 142 (2):513–516
15. Domingo C, Pomares X (2013) Can omalizumab be effective in chronic eosinophilic pneumonia? Chest 143(1):274
16. Mukherjee M, Sehmi R, Nair P (2014) Anti-IL5 therapy for asthma and beyond. World Allergy Organ J 7(1):32
17. Lim HF, Nair P (2015) Efficacy and safety of reslizumab in patients with moderate to severe eosinophilic asthma. Expert Rev Respir Med 9(2):135–142
18. Varricchi G, Bagnasco D, Borriello F, Heffler E, Canonica GW (2016) Interleukin-5 pathway inhibition in the treatment of eosinophilic respiratory disorders: evidence and unmet needs. Curr Opin Allergy Clin Immunol 16(2):186
19. Pavord ID, Korn S, Howarth P, Bleecker ER, Buhl R, Keene ON, Ortega H, Chanez P (2012) Mepolizumab for severe eosinophilic asthma (DREAM): a multicentre, double-blind, placebo-controlled trial. Lancet 380(9842):651–659

20. Liu Y, Zhang S, Li DW, Jiang SJ (2013) Efficacy of anti-interleukin-5 therapy with mepolizumab in patients with asthma: a meta-analysis of randomized placebo-controlled trials. PLoS One 8(3):e59872
21. Garrett JK, Jameson SC, Thomson B, Collins MH, Wagoner LE, Freese DK, Beck LA, Boyce JA, Filipovich AH, Villanueva JM, Sutton SA, Assa'ad AH, Rothenberg ME (2004) Anti-interleukin-5 (mepolizumab) therapy for hypereosinophilic syndromes. J Allergy Clin Immunol 113(1):115–119
22. Sarkis E, Patel S, Burns K, Batarseh H, Mador MJ (2020) Anti-interleukin (IL)-5 as a steroid-sparing agent in chronic eosinophilic pneumonia. J Asthma 57:82–86
23. To M, Kono Y, Yamawaki S, Soeda S, Katsube O, Kishi H, To Y (2018) A case of chronic eosinophilic pneumonia successfully treated with mepolizumab. J Allergy Clin Immunol Pract 6(5):1746
24. Castro M (2018) Dupilumab efficacy and safety in moderate-to-severe uncontrolled asthma. N Engl J Med 378(26):2486–2496
25. Naughton M, Fahy J, FitzGerald MK (1993) Chronic eosinophilic pneumonia: a long-term follow-up of 12 patients. Chest 103(1):162–165
26. Durieu J, Wallaert B, Tonnel A (1997) Long-term follow-up of pulmonary function in chronic eosinophilic pneumonia. Groupe d'Etude en Pathologie Interstitielle de la Societe de PathologieThoracique du Nord. Eur Respir J 10(2):286–291
27. Hauswaldt J, Blaschke S (2017) [Dyspnea]. Internist (Berl) 58(9):925–936
28. Berliner D, Schneider N, Welte T, Bauersachs J (2016) The differential diagnosis of dyspnea. Dtsch Arztebl Int 113(49):834–845
29. Sattar SBA, Sharma S (2019) Bacterial pneumonia. StatPearls Publishing, Treasure Island, FL
30. Falcone M, Venditti M, Shindo Y, Kollef MH (2011) Healthcare-associated pneumonia: diagnostic criteria and distinction from community-acquired pneumonia. Int J Infect Dis 15 (8):e545–e550
31. Grief SN, Loza JK (2018) Guidelines for the evaluation and treatment of pneumonia. Prim Care 45(3):485–503
32. Franquet T (2018) Imaging of community-acquired pneumonia. J Thorac Imaging 33 (5):282–294
33. Anand N, Kollef MH (2009) The alphabet soup of pneumonia: CAP, HAP, HCAP, NHAP, and VAP. Semin Respir Crit Care Med 30(1):3–9
34. Rayees S, Mabalirajan U, Bhat WW, Rasool S, Rather RA, Panda L, Satti NK, Latoo SK, Ghosh B, Singh G (2015) Therapeutic effects of R8, a semi-synthetic analogue of Vasicine, on murine model of allergic airway inflammation via STAT6 inhibition. Int Immunopharmacol 26 (1):246–256

Tuberculosis

5

Shipra Bhatt, Abhishek Gour, Gurdarshan Singh, and Utpal Nandi

Abstract

Tuberculosis (TB) is one of the lethal diseases that affect millions of people around the world. The primary concern associated with this endemic ailment is an elevated level of resistance. World Health Organisation (WHO) has taken steps to reduce the incidence of TB at an accelerated rate under the purview of ending the TB epidemic by 2030. To achieve this goal, there are hurdles that need to be addressed, which are not only limited to TB diagnosis, treatment, and prevention but also linked to dealing with social and economic determinants in close collaboration with diverse sectors in the healthcare domain. In this scenario, this chapter focuses on the epidemiology of TB, primary causes and symptoms of TB, pathophysiological process of TB along with the involvement of cells and transcriptional factors, current treatment regimen with its drawbacks, and future treatment options. This chapter represents an up-to-date overview of these disease conditions and its therapy in global perspectives.

Keywords

Tuberculosis · Epidemiology · Pathophysiology · Drug resistance · Antitubercular drugs

S. Bhatt · A. Gour · G. Singh · U. Nandi (✉)
PK-PD, Toxicology and Formulation Division, CSIR-Indian Institute of Integrative Medicine, Jammu, Jammu & Kashmir, India

Academy of Scientific and Innovative Research (AcSIR), CSIR-Indian Institute of Integrative Medicine, Jammu, Jammu & Kashmir, India
e-mail: unandi@iiim.ac.in

S. Rayees et al. (eds.), *Chronic Lung Diseases*,
https://doi.org/10.1007/978-981-15-3734-9_5

Abbreviations

ART	Antiretroviral therapy
ATP	Adenosine triphosphate
BCG	Bacillus Calmette–Guerin
DIM	Dimycocerosate phthiocerol;
DOT	Directly observed therapy
DOTS	Directly observed treatment, short-course
HIV	Human immunodeficiency virus
ILC	Innate lymphoid cells
LAM	Lipoarabinomannan
LTBI	Latent tuberculosis infection
MAIT	Mucosa-associated invariant T
Man-LAM	Mannose capped lipoarabinomannan
MDR	Multidrug resistance
MIC	Minimum inhibitory concentration
Mtb	*Mycobacterium tuberculosis*
NAA	Nucleic acid amplification
PIM	Phosphatidylinositol mannoside
PLGA	Poly lactide-co-glycolide
RD-1	Region of difference-1
RR	Rifampicin resistant
SL	Sulfated glycolipid
TB	Tuberculosis
TDM	Trehalose dimycolates
TST	Tuberculosis skin test
USFDA	United States Food and Drug Administration
WHO	World Health Organization
XDR	Extremely drug resistance

5.1 Introduction

TB is one of the life-threatening communicable diseases caused by different species of *Mycobacterium*. Humans have probably been suffering from this infection since the Neolithic period [1]. It is one of the leading causes of death and considered as a key health burden in both developing and developed countries. As per the WHO report 2019, approximately ten million people have been suffering from TB globally, out of which the majority of individuals were men. The pathogen can invade the alveoli of lungs, and then, it is engulfed by macrophages. The capability to survive inside the macrophages, host-defense mechanism destruction, and manipulation in phagosome maturation determine the success of pathogen within the host [2]. Although effective treatment options are available for TB, an increasing concern of resistance to the existing therapy in the form of multidrug resistance (MDR) and extensively drug resistance (XDR) leads to a high mortality rate. The emerging resistant strains of *Mycobacterium tuberculosis (Mtb)* give emphasis to the need for the development of new antimycobacterial agents [3]. In the midst of the variety of treatment options against TB, nanoparticles and antitubercular therapeutic peptides emerge as leading alternatives for the management of this disease. Currently, the incidence of TB is declining at about 2% per year. There is a need to achieve a 4–5% yearly decline to attain 2020 milestone of the End TB Strategy. Between 2000 and 2018, about 58 million lives were protected via its diagnosis and treatment. The Sustainable Development Goals regarding health targets have important criteria to end the TB endemic by 2030 [4].

5.1.1 About the Disease

Mycobacterium has been believed to be originated over 150 million years ago. *Mycobacterium ulcerans* is the pathogen for TB-causing infection since ancient times [5]. Early hominids from the region of east Africa have been infected by *Mtb* about 3 million years ago [6]. The initial documents related to TB were found in India and China about 3300 and 2300 years ago, respectively [7, 8]. Archaeological evidence by Peruvian mummies demonstrated that Pott's deformities were still there before the immigration of the European pioneers of South America in the Andean region [9–11]. At the beginning of the twentieth century, increasing air pollution, increasing population, and crowded working conditions might have detrimental effects on the transmission of TB in some instances [12]. The recent members of *Mycobacterium* complex include *Mtb* and also its African variants *Mycobacterium africanum*, *Mycobacterium canettii*, and *Mycobacterium bovis*, which had a common African predecessor about 35,000–15,000 years ago [6, 13]. Franciscus Sylvius observed that phthisis was accompanied by tubercles. In 1679, he coined the term "tubercula" (small knots) that means lung nodules [14]. Benjamin Marten in 1722 was the first to speculate the infectious nature of the disease. According to him, TB was caused by "animalculae or their seed inimicable to our Nature," and these spread through a breath that discharges from lungs and can be trapped by a healthy individual. In 1865, Jean-Antoine Villemin demonstrated that TB was communicable by transferring fluid as well as pus cells from bovine and human lesions to rabbits, which ultimately develop TB. The finding was discredited by Koch later on. In 1882, he isolated *Mtb* from crushed tubercles and cultured them [15]. According to Koch's postulates: "To demonstrate that TB is caused by the invasion of bacilli and conditioned by the growth and multiplication of bacilli but it was necessary: (1) to isolate the bacilli from the body; (2) grow them in pure culture; and (3) by administering the isolated bacilli to animals, reproduce the same morbid condition." According to Koch's experiment, the re-inoculation of animals with bacilli after several weeks resulted in the production of merely a definite red nodule that ultimately healed, which demonstrate the presence of immunity toward infection. In 1890, he announced that disease is healed by the culture filtrates, which were discredited. Later, those filtrates were purified partially and became the principle of the tuberculin skin test (TST) [15, 16]. Koch also contributed for explanation of the infectious etiology of TB for which he got a Nobel Prize in Medicine in 1905 [9, 17]. Before the availability of an effective treatment regimen for TB, its treatment involved isolation in sanatoria [12]. In 1854, Hermann Brehmer created the first sanatorium in Europe. He has a belief that altitude and exercise would help in treating TB [18]. Afterward, Brehmer found an institution in the region of Gorbersdorf, a peak area located in Fir forest to cure patients with constant clean and fresh air with healthy nutrition. Later, sanatoria were built and allowed for the curing of TB patients in the next 10 years. Its infectious nature was revealed by Jean-Antoine Villemin, a French military surgeon in 1865. He formulated his theory to scrutinize that TB was more common among soldiers who lived in barracks for long times than those who lived in the field [16]. The first sanatorium was established by Edward Livingston Trudeau in the United States in 1882. He instigated a public health movement that stresses on the outdoor life and ordinances to get better hygiene. Another treatment option involved pasteurization of cow's milk, thus declining the likelihood of infection by *Mycobacterium bovis*. Albert Calmette and Camille Guerin in 1908 tried to solve the issue of bacillary clumping linked to the pathogen by growing bacilli in a disseminated culture that enclosed bile of ox. In 39th passage, they observed a morphological variant that showed virulence in various animal species and provided a protective action against virulent *Mtb*. In 231st passage, this strain was given to a child whose mother died while giving birth. Bacillus Calmette–Guerin (BCG) vaccine is the extensively used vaccine. In 1947, antibiotics were introduced for the treatment of TB, although isoniazid was synthesized first in 1912, but took a long time to be used as an effective antitubercular drug. After that, introduction of *p*-aminosalicylic acid led to a dramatic reduction in mortality from TB. With this, the era of sanatorium ended [15]. In the 1990s, WHO developed and disseminated a new approach for controlling TB: directly observed treatment, short-course (DOTS) strategy [19]. According to DOTS strategy, there were five important elements for control of TB: government commitment; bacteriological diagnosis mainly in patients spontaneously seeking care at health centers; standardized short-course chemotherapy under proper case management conditions; an effective drug supply system, and a monitoring and evaluation system allowing assessment of notifications and treatment outcomes. In 1993, WHO declared TB as a global health emergency [20], and then, in 2006, WHO enhanced the DOTS strategy to combat new health challenges like human immunodeficiency virus (HIV)-associated TB and MDR-TB.

5.1.2 Epidemiology/Morbidity

The burden of TB disease can be considered in terms of incidence, prevalence, and mortality. Incidence is defined as the total number of new and relapse cases of TB that arise in a particular time frame, usually one year. Prevalence is the number of TB cases at a specified time period. Mortality is the total number of deaths in a particular time period, generally 1 year. Eighty-seven percent of the TB cases were reported from 30 high disease burden countries where two thirds of total cases were from eight countries, such as India, China, Pakistan, Bangladesh, the Philippines, Nigeria, Indonesia, and South Africa. On the contrary, about 6% of total cases are in the European and American regions of WHO. Chances for the development of active TB disease are extremely high in infants as compared to children of age group 2–10 years. The possibility of disease development increases during adolescence and rises near the age of 25 years and remains persistent throughout life. Worldwide, the proportions of TB incidence were 64% in males and 36% were in females. The male-to-female ratio of TB incidence for different age groups varied from 1.3 to 2.1 in the WHO region of Eastern Mediterranean and Western Pacific. In children, it was close to 1.

HIV infection is one of the most influential risk factors for active TB disease as chances of TB infections are around 20 times more in HIV-positive individuals than in the rest of the population. This disease was one of the principal causes of hospitalization in HIV-infected children and adults. Approximately 23% of the world's population has latent TB infection, and they are at high risk of progressing active TB disease. International Classification of Diseases determines the TB mortality among HIV-negative individuals. If an HIV-positive individual dies from TB infection, the cause of death is considered to be as HIV. Among HIV-negative individuals, the WHO region of Africa and South East Asia has witnessed 82% mortality rate and India had 32%, and also, these regions reported for 85% of total TB deaths among HIV-positive and HIV-negative individuals, where India had 27%. About 1.3 million people had died because of TB among HIV-negative patients, and three million additional deaths occurred in patients suffering from HIV infection. The percentage of individuals who died with TB had reduced from 23% to 16% from 2000 to 2017. Worldwide, the number of TB deaths among HIV-negative individuals has reduced from 29% to 5%, and in the case of HIV-positive individuals, the number has reduced from 44% to 20% from 2000 to 2015. In HIV-negative individuals, the mortality rate is decreasing 3% per year from 2000 to 2017. The rate of incidence of TB was decreased by 1.8% from 2016 to 2017.

One of the significant threats to public health is drug-resistant TB, where the emergence of drug resistance and its distribution are heterogeneous. About 5.6 million individuals have developed rifampicin-resistant TB (RR-TB), 82% possessed MDR-TB, and 8.5% have XDR-TB. Nearly, half of the global cases of MDR/RR-TB were found in three countries, of which 24% were from India, followed by China, and then the Russian Federation. Worldwide, MDR-TB prevalence is approximately 5%. However, it fluctuates from 1% to 20% in different countries. In China, one fourth of the patients suffering from TB have developed resistance toward isoniazid or rifampicin, while India has observed the appearance of totally drug-resistant strains. There were approximately five million incident cases of MDR/RR-TB in 2017. Countries such as Ukraine, Pakistan, Azerbaijan, Bangladesh, Belarus, and South Africa have developed resistance to first-line drugs that were 19% for new cases and 43% for already treated cases.

The percentage of individuals who die from TB disease is expressed in terms of the case fatality ratio. It is represented as the ratio of the number of deaths to the total number of new cases in a particular year. It permits the evaluation of difference inequity in provisions for accessing the diagnosis and treatment of TB among countries. To achieve the goal of End TB Strategy, the fatality ratio needs to reduce to 10% and 6.5% by 2020 and 2025, respectively. It was reduced from 23% to 16% from 2000 to 2017. In 2017, MDR/RR-TB was found in approximately 3.5% of fresh and 18% of previously treated cases that lead to the death of two million patients.

The Sustainable Development Goals have set the target to decline TB incidence and mortality rate by 20% and 35%, respectively, at set milestone by 2020. In the subsequent phase, set the target by 2030 for the reduction in TB incidence and mortality rate to 80% and 90%, respectively. A further target is to decline in TB incidence and mortality rate by 90% and 95%, respectively, by 2035 [21].

5.1.3 Causes/Symptoms

TB is a potentially severe infectious disease that is primarily caused by *Mtb*. Other species that are responsible for TB infection include *Mycobacterium canettii*, *Mycobacterium africanum*, *Mycobacterium microti*, *Mycobacterium bovis*, etc. [22]. *Mtb* is an actinomycete that shows close relation to saprophytic bacteria like *Mycobacterium smegmatis*. Unlike most Gram-positive bacteria, the peptidoglycan wall of these bacilli is augmented with an arrangement of complex lipidoglycans, which protects them from desiccation in soil. Approximately 30% of genes in these bacteria is responsible for the synthesis or metabolism of lipids. These preadaptations like thick waxy cell wall and the capability to catabolize fatty acids appear to be useful for parasitic existence [23]. *Mtb* spreads via minute airborne droplets (droplet nuclei) which are generated while talking, coughing, and sneezing by a patient suffering from laryngeal or pulmonary TB. These droplet nuclei can suspend in the air for several minutes to hours past expectoration [24]. There are a number of factors that influence the transmission of the bacteria, such as number and virulence of bacilli in the droplets, degree of exposure to air, event of aerosolization, and exposure of bacilli toward UV light. *Mtb* introduction into the lungs causes infection in the respiratory tract; however, this infection can transmit to other sites of the body, such as the lymphatic system, pleura, bones/joints, or meninges, and it is termed as extrapulmonary TB [25].

TB may progress in a different way in patients on the basis of the immune system. Stages of disease progression include latency, primary disease, primary progressive disease, and extrapulmonary disease. Each stage is marked by distinct manifestations. Different types of TB and its symptoms are described.

Latent TB infection (LTBI): Persons with latent TB do not feel illness having no signs and symptoms of TB [26]. However, bacilli can stay alive in the necrotic matter for several years or up to existence where the disease may be reactivated in the immunocompromised conditions [27]. However, co-infection with HIV is the prominent reason for the development of active disease and other factors like malnutrition, smoking, sepsis, diabetes mellitus, chemotherapy, organ transplantation, and renal failure. All these factors contribute toward the reactivation of the remote infection [28, 26].

Primary disease: Primary TB is most frequently asymptomatic, and thus, the only evidence of the disease is the resulted form of diagnostic tests. Paratracheal lymphadenopathy arises as the bacteria transmit to the lymphatic system from the lungs. The swelling of lesions leads to pleural effusion as the bacilli disseminate within the pleural space from an adjacent site. The developed effusion can grow too large to stimulate other symptoms such as pleuritic chest pain, fever, and dyspnea.

Primary progressive TB: Around 10% of individuals who are exposed to bacilli develop this infection. Early signs and symptoms are mostly uncertain but observed during progression toward an active form of the disease. Disease symptoms are majorly exhaustion, malaise, and mild fever, along with chills and night sweats [25]. Wasting, a characteristic facet of the disease, involves the loss of fat and lean tissue; fatigue may result due to decrease in muscle mass or loss of appetite or altered metabolism [29]. Finger clubbing may take place, which is the delayed response toward lack of oxygen, although this is not the indication for the extent of disease [30]. Cough develops in most of the patients, though it may be nonproductive in the beginning, but eventually, it can lead to cough with purulent sputum with some streaks of blood. Rupture of a dilated vessel in the wall of the cavity, destruction of a patent vessel, or the synthesis of an aspergilloma in the old cavity can lead to hemoptysis. The inflammation in the parenchyma may lead to pleuritic chest pain. An increase in the interstitial volume can cause a reduction in the diffusion capacity of lungs, which may lead to dyspnea or orthopnea [25].

Extrapulmonary TB: Pulmonary system is the most common location for the disease. During the initial pulmonary infection, *Mtb* potentially infects almost every organ through lymphohematogenous dissemination. In the case of patients with acquired immunodeficiency syndrome, extrapulmonary TB is considered as a diagnostic criterion. Immunocompromised persons show an increased risk of developing this disease. Depending on the affected site, extrapulmonary tuberculosis can be of various types such as lymphatic TB, miliary TB, and TB of central nervous system [31]. The pleural cavity is one of the sites where TB infection can take place. In the pleural space, the rupturing of small subpleural focus leads to TB pleural effusion. This causes communication between the bacilli and their particular components that leads to a delayed type of hypersensitivity reaction. Symptoms may include pleuritic chest pain and high fever; however, the most common symptoms are chronic pleuritis with pain, low-grade fever, progressive dyspnea, dry cough, and asthenia. The most common type of extrapulmonary TB is lymph node TB, where *Mtb* affects the peripheral lymph node chain. In the supraclavicular and cervical region, a distinct painless swelling develops. The progression of the disease may lead to fistulas. In this case, unrelated systemic symptoms appear, suspicion of an immunodepressive disease or HIV infection is to be supposed, and cervical adenopathy occurs most often [32]. Another type of extrapulmonary TB is genitourinary TB. Frequently accounted symptoms are dysuria, pollakiuria, hematuria, and flank pain. In women, genital TB can give rise to infertility, menstrual abnormalities, and pelvic pain. In men, it can lead to prostatitis and orchitis, or it can affect epididymis, forming a slightly painful mass [33]. In case of bone TB, the most affected sites are spine, hips, and knees. The major symptom in this situation is pain. It may lead to swelling in peripheral joints [34]. The most harmful site where the infection can spread is the central nervous system, which may cause meningitis or space-occupying tuberculomas, which are followed by headache, anorexia, general malaise, neck rigidity, decreased consciousness, and vomiting. If the disease spreads to the brain parenchyma, it results in convulsions and focal signs. Tubercular meningitis is fatal in most cases if timely treatment is not provided [28]. Laryngeal tuberculosis is the most common granulomatous disease of the larynx. Symptoms include the change in voice, aphonia, and irritation in throat. Pulmonary TB is always associated with laryngeal TB [35]. Another form of extrapulmonary TB is miliary TB, caused by the hematogenous transmission of *Mtb*. In miliary TB, lesions are of constant size, having the size less than 2 mm like millet seed. Other common symptoms include loss of weight, night sweats, anorexia, and fever [36, 37].

5.2 Pathophysiology of TB

5.2.1 Biology of the Disease

Mtb is the most common species among all *Mycobacterium*, which is responsible for TB infection. The bacterial infection is transmitted in the form of droplets having a diameter of 1–5 μm hovering in the air during coughing, speaking, or sneezing of the person with active TB. The environment and extent of exposure, the infectiousness of TB source, and the immune system of an individual are the essential factors that determine the likelihood of transmission of infection to another individual. The airborne infectious droplets come close to the terminal airspaces by inhalation and then infect the alveolar macrophages. Age, intravenous drug administration, recent TB infection, immunodeficiency ensuing from HIV infection, immunosuppressant drugs, and transplantation of organs are the important characteristics allied with an increased risk of progression of active TB. Among all, the strongest acknowledged risk factor for emergent active TB is HIV infection [22]. Patients who undergo tumor necrosis factor-alpha inhibitor therapy are at higher risk of reactivation, and there is a continuous need to access TB in these patients by radiologist. Diabetes mellitus, chronic renal failure, silicosis, low body weight, alcohol or tobacco abuse, prior gastrectomy or jejunoileal bypass, and malignancies like leukemia, head, neck, and lung carcinoma are the conditions that augment the risk of active TB [38].

The word “Granuloma” was first used by Rudolph Virchow in 1818 to illustrate tumor that ulcerate and give rise to granulation tissue [39, 40]. It is defined as the assortment of inflammatory cells dominated by mononuclear cells and also involves a large figure of enzymes and cytokines [41]. Imperative research precedence is interpreting the underlying mechanism involving granulomas maintenance, which is associated with control of infection and persistence of the *Mtb* [42]. From host viewpoint, granuloma has the ability to wall off contagion from the body, so-called bacterial prison. From bacterial viewpoint, it is an increasing assortment of phagocytic cells to transmit disease and multiply inside the host. The recruitment of developing granuloma of myeloid cells is highly permissive to *Mtb* infection due to secretion system ESX-1 from the region of difference 1 (RD-1) that initiates the type-1 interferon response [43]. RD1 contains genes of bacterial secretion system ESX-1, which is responsible for the release of bacterial product into the cytoplasm of macrophages when bacteria undergo phagocytosis [44]. This secretion system plays a vital role in the pathogenesis of active TB. A few non-TB mycobacteria like *Mycobacterium kansasii* and *Mycobacterium marinum* also possess a conserved ESX-1 antigen that has encouraged a reconsideration of the ability of ESX-1 in the virulence of *Mtb* [45]. So, it is necessary to consider but not exclusively liable for the virulence of *Mtb* [46]. Immune responses are segregated in the region of the granulomas having proinflammatory cells constituent at its center and anti-inflammatory in neighboring tissue [47]. Granuloma shows some extent of variation in its pattern of organization. The essential constituents of granulomas are macrophages, which are predominated centrally, and their function is to remove the pathogen via phagocytosis. The activated macrophages possess an abundant, pale, eosinophilic cytoplasm so that adjacent macrophages form a continuous sheet, parallel to the surface epithelium due to indistinct margins and are called as epithelioid cells and granuloma is called as epithelioid cell granuloma. These cells fuse to form a multinucleated giant cell. There are two types of giant cells in TB. One is the Langhans type in which nuclei are organized in the periphery, and the cytoplasm is at the center and exhibited a rosette-like structure [48]. Other is the foreign-body type of giant cells where nuclei do not show regular arrangements. In immunological-induced granulomas, lymphocytes cells are more prominent. Eosinophils are other types of inflammatory cells that form the granuloma. The entire granuloma undergoes fibrosis, hyalinization, calcification, and even ossification, indicating the presence of necrosis in the center. The histopathological abrasion of TB is the example of a necrotizing epithelioid cell granuloma [49]. Galen observed tubercles in various animals (tubercle, Latin tuberculum—a diminutive of a tuber, small swelling) in the condition known as hydrops thoracis.

Mtb has numerous adaptive strategies to endure within host macrophages by destructing the phagosome pathways [50]. Bacterial cell wall possesses varied lipid contents such as sulfated glycolipid (SL), dimycocerosate phthiocerol (DIM), trehalose dimycolates (TDM), mannose capped lipoarabinomannan (Man-LAM), lipoarabinomannan (LAM), and phosphatidylinositol mannoside (PIM) that contribute to its virulent activity. PIM and LAM apprehend the fusion of phagosomes and acidification, thereby hindering the phagosome pathway [51, 52]. TDM and SL check the lysosomes fusion [53]. DIM contributes toward the development of permeability barriers and inhibition of acidification [54]. Several factors are evident to render individuals susceptible to or associated with high chances of TB, resulting in a decrease in immunity [55].

Primary TB is a disease caused by *Mtb* in a person having no previous exposure to infection. Recent research in the field of TB has revealed that granulomas are the vital abrasion in both types of TB. The most primitive basis of primary TB was laid by Marie-Jules Parrot in 1876. When the perceptive of TB was based on several assumptions, primary TB was explained in terms of the Parrot law, which states that "pulmonary TB does not exist in the child without the involvement of the tracheobronchial gland." In 1896, George Kuss states that pathology of TB was due to aerogenous infection, which is understood as primary TB in his monograph. But his thoughts did not get much attention. In 1907, Eugene Albrecht extended the concept of primary TB from childhood to adult TB, and Hans Albrecht in 1909 established the interpretation of Kuss and convoluted on Parrot law. This work created the bases of the examination of Anton Ghon [56]. Primary TB defends the host by the production of effectual systemic immunity to check disseminated infection. It is an infection that arises with an inadequate person's immunity, which restricts and manages pathogens in granulomas. It produces a variety of infection states that vary from disseminated TB in persons with HIV, miliary TB, and pulmonary granulomas that arise characteristically in extremely young, immunologically naive, old, and in immunosuppressed persons. The infection can spread to lymph nodes via lymphatics or the bloodstream and other organs too. This infection can be controlled within weeks, and the abrasion heals in the immunocompetent group. Primary TB protects the individual effectively from dissemination via the production of systemic immunity, which has become the "central dogma" of immunity mediated through granulomas, macrophages, and production of IFN-γ. Lesions of primary TB can reappear when immunosuppression decreases T-cell-mediated immunity. In primary TB, there is a unit encompassing the focus and infected lymph nodes, identified as the primary complex of the Ranke, which consists of intervening lymphatics between the lesion and the lymph nodes. The center of primary infection in the lung is generally subpleural, in the middle portion of the lower lobe or lower portion of the middle lobe, called Ghon's focus. Therefore, the unit of Ghon's focus and the draining tracheobronchial lymph nodes is the Ghon's complex [57].

Postprimary TB characteristically commences only after primary TB and generally arises due to endogenous reactivation, that is, in a person who is previously exposed to bacterial infection. Postprimary TB produces cavities where pathogen undergoes multiple divisions and finally escapes to the environment by evading and distorting systemic immunity. A little is known about the mechanisms behind the pathology of postprimary TB. The bacteria, by some mean influence the host for early penetration and are able to survive in alveolar macrophages. The bronchioles ensnared the mycobacterial antigen and lipids in the region of alveolar macrophages and finally get obstructed. The infiltration gradually extends through bronchi and to the other region of the lung. It can revert or go through necrosis to turn into caseous pneumonia to produce cavities through fragmentation or may retain to develop into the focus of fibrocaseous disease [58]. Patients having immune responses measured via TST are the ones who are most likely to develop clinical disease. It was described by most of the pathologists via X-rays in preantibiotic era. In 1920s, it was known as Assmann's focus regarded as the appearance of "raisin on a stem." In 1990s, CT scans displayed better and coined the word "tree-in-bud," indicating the distinctive characteristics of pulmonary TB. In recent years, it has been long established by using CT and PET-CT in South Africa and Latvia [59–61]. The location of postprimary TB is apical and subapical, and by Medlar, this area is considered to be a vulnerable region [62].

Pulmonary TB was evident with four distinctive phases ensuing mycobacterial infection. Each of these phases is indomitable by the homeostasis between bacillary factors and the immune system of the host [63]. Following inhalation of pathogen, alveolar macrophages ingest the bacterial pathogens and destroy them through phagocytosis. Bacilli continue to divide by evading initial destruction by phagocytosis. The ability of macrophages to destroy the pathogen depends on their intrinsic microbicidal capacity. The second phase is manifested by the logarithmic phase representing the growth of the pathogen within host. It is characterized by the recruitment of monocytes and other inflammatory cells to the lungs. Monocytes differentiate into macrophages but fail to eliminate the pathogen. The pathological sites are accompanied by antigen-specific T cells that activate the monocytoid cells, which undergo differentiation into giant cells, epithelioid cells, and multinucleated Langhans cells. This is a third stage characterized by granuloma formation, preventing the propagation of bacilli and walling off the infection from infected person. This stage of latency disturbs under conditions of falling immune surveillance followed by endogenous reactivation of infection characterized by the termination of necrosis.

5.2.2 Cell Types Involved in TB

The stability between the bacilli and the magnitude of the immune response is elicited by host maintained through protective immunity against the pathogen. Numerous immune system cells are involved not only to eliminate the bacterial infection but also to maintain the steady-state control over the spread and prevention of the disease concerning granuloma formation. An innate and adaptive immune response is involved as antitubercular immunity at various levels throughout infection.

The primary defensive barrier against pathogen is respiratory tract epithelial cells [64]. Nonhematopoietic epithelial cells play a vital role in defense by secreting antimicrobial molecules, enzymes, peptides, cytokines, chemokines, and growth factors. All these molecules lead to the commencement of innate immune response that is significant in control of infection [65, 66]. Airway epithelial cells are the primitive cells encountering pathogen after inhalation and play an important role in the recognition and internalization of the pathogen after its binding within the host [67]. These cells possess pattern recognition receptors like RIG-1, TLRs, NOD, and C-type lectins, additionally, surfactant's proteins that attach to cell wall of the pathogen [68–70]. Upon recognition, pathogen stimulates the cytokines, including GM-CSF, IFN-γ, TNF-α, IL-6, IL-10, and chemokines, such as MCP-1, IP-10, IL-8, IL-27 [71–75], via activation of signaling pathways, thus leading to activation of various cell types including phagocytes, lymphocytes, and polymorphonuclear leukocytes to the pulmonary region [76]. These epithelial cells play a vital function in the production of adaptive immunity toward infection by expressing major histocompatibility complex-1 molecules and, thus, stimulating IFN-γ production [77]. These cells possess both innate and adaptive immunity against pathogens throughout infection. In a case study, it has been found that the introduction of a pathogen cannot lead to infection at all times. In epidemic area, in TST, half of the exposed individuals certainly do not get infected and become negative to the test, and in the IFN-γ release test, half of the individuals remain positive due to lack of Th1-type adaptive immunity against pathogen [78].

Neutrophils are the primary immune cells having a significant role in the innate and acute inflammatory response [79]. These cells produce antimicrobial enzymes, such as matrix metalloproteases, lactoferrin, α-defensins, and lipocalin, which limit the survival of pathogen within phagocytic cells followed by phagocytosis, thereby restraining the survival of pathogen. Upon stimulation, they secrete chemokines and proinflammatory cytokines to elicit the immune responses [80]. Natural killer cells are a well-known cellular component of innate immunity that act through the production of different cytokines [81, 82]. In acute infection, these cells possess increased cytotoxicity, production of IFN-γ and TNF-α, and upregulation of NKD2D/NKp46 [83–85]. They exhibit lysis of infected macrophages, monocytes, and pathogen-expanded T regulatory cells, thus inducing the production of γδ-T cell and IFN-γ [86, 87]. These cells possess low cytotoxicity, less IFN-γ production, and reduced expression of NKp30 and NKp46 in a patient affected with active TB [88, 89]. Natural killer T cells are the cells expressing both natural killer cells and T-cell markers having effector and regulatory functions [90, 91]. These cells provide protection against TB infection in both mouse and human models [92]. It has been found that patient with active TB possesses dysfunctional natural killer cells with augmented expression of inhibitory agent, that is, PD-1 [93]. Another study displayed that natural killer cells during ex vivo antigen stimulation secrete TNF-α, IFN-γ, IL-17, IL-2, and IL-21 [94, 95]. T-regulatory cells are a unique type of T cell that exhibit $CD4^+$ cells expressing CD25 to suppress the other T cells via contact-dependent and contact-independent cytokine-mediated pathways. They are recruited at the infectious site via CCR1 and CCR4 chemokine receptors and secrete IL-10 and TGF-β that exhibit a suppressive effect on activated T cells [96]. γδ T cells provide primary protection against pulmonary TB and form a linkage between innate and adaptive immunity. These cells are recruited to the infectious site in the early phase of infection and induce IFN-γ and IL-17 [97]. The frequencies of these cells are increased at the lungs in active TB [98]. Mucosa-associated invariant T (MAIT) cells originate from thymus and are prevalent mostly in the blood as well as mucosal sites in humans. These cells are secreted during stimulation by vitamin B metabolites found in bacteria and elicit an immune response via cytokine production like IFN-γ and TNF-α and also produce cytotoxic granules liable for cell lysis [99, 100]. Due to the absence of MAIT cells in mice, the mycobacterial load is higher upon infection [101]. MAIT cells migrate to infectious site from periphery. Thus, the frequency of these cells in infected individual is significantly reduced in peripheral blood, but a higher number is available in the lungs [102]. Innate lymphoid cells (ILC) have emerged from an ID-2-dependent lymphoid progenitor cell that exhibits the first line of defense against pathogen and immune homeostasis. These cells have exhibited to elicit the barrier function between epithelium of lungs and tissue homeostasis in the area of the respiratory tract [103]. On the basis of expression of surface markers, effector cytokines, and transcription factor, there are three types, namely ILC1, ILC2, and ILC3, that exhibit phenotypic and functional heterogeneity [104]. They have appeared as a new member of the innate counterparts of T-helper lymphocytes. It has been found that ILC population significantly decreased in drug-susceptible and drug-resistant TB infection. The level of ILC1 and ILC3 was restored during the treatment of drug-susceptible TB but not ILC2. ILC population displays a high level of CD69, CD25, and CCR6 (activation markers). These findings revealed that the intonation of ILC population possibly has a pathogenic and defensive role during infection. These cells possibly shape the victory and letdown of *Mtb* for causing a long-term infection via active adaptive immunity [105]. The interaction of the pathogen with different cell types such as epithelial cells, endothelial cells, adipocytes, and neurons frequently elicit immune response to conquer the disease conditions [106]. It has been found that the effect of drugs in a patient with MDR-TB was enhanced by daily low-dose administration of recombinant IL-2 due to immune system activation [107]. There is a need for implementation of a new strategy by changing the chemokines and cytokines balance so as to modulate the immune response. Administration of heat-killed preparation of other mycobacteria along with chemotherapy could enhance the immune response [108]. Immunopotentiation with adjuvant therapeutic vaccination exhibits an improved Th1 immunity in an infected patient. Thalidomide and pentoxifylline have been found to save the patient via inhibition of TNF-α. Levamisole is widely used in TB because of its action as IL-2 and IFN-γ inhibitor [109].

5.2.3 Transcriptional Regulations

Antibiotics have the potential to activate or inhibit the gene expression in bacteria. Gene expression profile can provide information about a pathogen and its capability to escape from the effect of antibiotics. Further, these also assist in scrutinizing the functioning of the pathogen during drug treatments. Transcriptional response in *Mycobacterium* toward antibiotics consists of the whole-genome array to access the effect of various types of drugs, drugs in combination, and growth factors [110]. It also permits access to the genes that are differentially expressed in both drug-sensitive and drug-resistant isolates. Thus, profiling of genes possibly will become a novel strategy for improving the efficacy of drugs. The drugs are classified based on the mechanism of action like inhibitors of DNA gyrase, translation, transcription, or cell wall biosynthesis. Drugs like isoniazid, ethionamide, thiolactomycin, and cerulenin display a similar type of expression, that is, inhibition of fatty acid and mycolic acid synthesis, with Kas operon induction (acpM-kasA-kasB-accD6), thus, encoding fatty acid synthase enzyme in the FAS II system and efpA gene that encodes for efflux transporters [111]. Pretomanid (PA-824) acts on bacterial cell wall as well as on respiratory complexes. During phase-III clinical trial, pretomanid displayed accumulation of methylglyoxal, a toxic metabolite which is responsible for the action [112]. Chelerythrine, a natural compound isolated from roots of *Chelidonium majus*, exhibits antimycobacterial activity via inhibition of translation. Upon treatment with this compound, there is a reduced expression of gene Rv0467 encoding an enzyme, namely isocitrate lyase, that mediates the conversion of isocitrate into succinate and glyoxylate, which is needed for growth and virulence of *Mtb* [113, 114]. Capreomycin, a peptide produced by *Streptomyces capreolus*, binds to 16S rRNA and 23S rRNA for inhibition of protein synthesis. Despite their role in inhibition of protein synthesis, it also activates the genes that encode Rv2416c and Rv1988, which promote the survival of pathogen inside the macrophages [115]. Linezolid, an antibiotic from the class of oxazolidinone, inhibits translation via binding to ribosomal subunit. It regulates the expression of 729 genes, which are involved in virulence, cell wall permeability, protein synthesis, and sulfite metabolism [116, 117]. Kanamycin, a second-line drug for the management of MDR-TB, interferes with protein synthesis by binding to 30S subunit of ribosome. It is evident from the literature that around 98 genes are upregulated and 198 genes are downregulated during its treatment [118]. The upregulated genes exhibit a variety of functional role like virulence, cell wall, and cellular processes, and PE/PPE family and downregulated ones are responsible for the metabolism of lipids [119]. Ra3160 and Ra3161 are the upregulated genes responsible for the growth of pathogen under the stress-induced condition as well as antimycobacterial tolerance and are reactive to kanamycin [120]. Vancomycin, a member of the glycopeptide family, inhibits the production of peptidoglycan, a chief constituent of the bacterial cell wall [121]. Upon vancomycin treatment, there is an augmented expression of genes like Rv2623 and chaperons encoding genes (hsp and htpX) which mediate oxidative stress response. Rv2623 is acknowledged for controlling the growth of bacteria and switch to latency through the ATP-dependent pathway. Adjuvant therapy with an inhibitor of Rv1152, a negative regulator of vancomycin-responsive genes, is recommended due to its high minimum inhibitory concentration (MIC) [122, 123]. Cycloserine, ethambutol, and isoniazid promote the transcription of whiB2, a transcriptional regulator that interrupts the formation of the cell wall [124, 125]. β-lactam antibiotics inhibit the synthesis of peptidoglycan, thereby disrupting the biosynthesis of cell wall. *Mtb* is resistant to β-lactam via β-lactamases formation [126]. Bedaquiline (TMC-207) is a recently approved antitubercular drug to combat MDR-TB. It acts by inhibiting the ATP synthase of mycobacteria [127, 128]. The transcription factors like Rv0324 and Rv0880 have a crucial role in regulating the bedaquiline response. Bacteria become oversensitive to bedaquiline by an interruption in these two genes through knock out. It has been evident that inhibition of Rv0880 regulation possibly induces the killing of bacteria due to bedaquiline potentiated by pretomanid [129, 130]. AX-35 is an arylvinylpiperazine amide that activates the cydABCD operon and thus hinders the cytochrome. C oxidase activity of *Mtb* [110], where CydA and CydB encode for terminal oxidase and cydCD encodes for transporters required for oxidase assembly. Rifampicin, a first-line antitubercular drug, binds to the β-subunit of RNA polymerase and interferes with transcription. It has been demonstrated in the most patients that *Mtb* becomes resistant to rifampicin due to mutation in RpoB gene [131].

The transcriptomic response in resistant strains has been explored by profiling of genome expression. Gene expression in both drug-sensitive and drug-resistant strains is entirely different and shows a discrepancy among diverse clinical strains with stable drug resistance profile [132–134]. In MDR strains, genes like EsxG, EsxH, RpsA, ESX-1, and rpmI are upregulated and lipF, groES, and narG are downregulated. Among all, EsxG–EsxH is a considerable protein responsible for the virulence of bacterial infection [132]. It has been demonstrated that genes like emb for cell wall synthesis, rpl for protein synthesis, sig and rpoB for transcription are downregulated and genes involved in efflux transporters and transcriptional machinery for stress response are upregulated, thus upregulation of efflux pumps elicit expulsion of antibiotic drugs which possibly will lead to resistance for antitubercular drugs [135]. In another study regarding XDR-TB, it has been found that expression of ethA gene is downregulated due to mutation in a promoter region, not because of repression of transcription by ethR [136]. In two XDR strains, the transcriptional response toward the drugs like isoniazid, ethionamide, and rifampicin has been studied and found that about 92 drug resistant genes are overexpressed in these strains which involve regulatory genes like Rv3676 and SenX3–RegX3, MprA–MprB, MtrA–MtrB, two-component regulatory system [3, 133].

Resistance against bacteria develops via mutations within the gene [137]. There is the vast majority of genes that have been associated with resistance. Within these genes, two main mechanisms coupled with resistance of drugs are the modification of targets and a defective enzyme that catalyze the formation of active drugs from prodrug. The underlying mechanism behind the resistance is hindered by limitations in the drug susceptibility test [138]. The result for the phenotypic susceptibility test is dichotomous, that is, *Mtb* is either prone or resistant to drug dosage, and these tests are standardized for isoniazid, rifampicin, and ethambutol. But the genotypic test might be unsuccessful to recognize a mutation within a phenotypically resistant isolate. The mutation can be of three types like companion, causal, compensatory, or stepping-stone. Assays are designed to detect drug resistance based on causal mutation. Therefore, it is crucial to identify the specific mutation responsible for drug resistance. Current research work are going on to identify resistance-allied mutation as well as to determine drug resistance at a faster rate than drug susceptibility test. In this direction, whole genome sequencing approach along with routine diagnostic workflows can be beneficial to identify drug resistance early while eliminating the phenotypic drug susceptibility at the same time [139–142].

5.3 Current Treatment

Current treatment options for TB compose of different facets, which are described as follows.

BCG is developed from live strains of *Mycobacterium bovis* which is utilized as an attenuated vaccine to prevent TB infections; it was developed by Calmette and Guérin. In 1921, BCG was first administered to humans, and it is highly effective to treat the severe forms of TB. It is a widely used vaccine in the world and administrated to over three billion individuals, especially for routine newborn immunization [143]. The vaccine has active ingredients like antigen and also has small amounts of other ingredients like salts of potassium, sodium, magnesium, and nontoxic stabilizer, that is, glycerol. It is effective against severe forms of TB like TB meningitis in children. The use of BCG vaccine against TB has been encouraged by the United Nations International Children's Emergency Fund, WHO, and Scandinavian Red Cross Societies [144]. This vaccine is not often administrated to a person having age more than 16 years because it does not work appropriately. However, it is administrated to a person having age in between 16 and 35 who are at increased risk of TB infection in the course of their work like healthcare workers. Vaccination is done via injection in the upper arm of person and usually leaves a small scar at the site of injection [145]. It has been evident that the efficacy of the vaccine against TB is found to be up to 80% [146, 147]. The cause of this variability in its efficacy is not clearly understood. The efficacy of the vaccine in infants and children below the age 5 to protect from severe form of TB is found to be in the range of 50–80% [148]; thus in children, vaccination is associated with protection from *Mtb* [147]. Later on, it has been found that TB mortality and morbidity are high in children below the age 5; thus, BCG vaccination is considered to be invaluable in this age group [149]. Meta-analysis reveals that the phase of defense is usually up to 10 years as effectiveness of vaccine declines with time [150]. It is uncertain that the present vaccination treatment approaches contribute toward the management of TB epidemic, as it is administrated at birth and improbably extends its defense to the stage of adolescence [151].

The currently available vaccine has possessed a protective immunity against TB, although the exact mechanism behind it is not well illuminated. This current regimen is focused on the prevention of active TB disease from rising in infected persons who cannot hold illness on their own as LTBI. A vaccine possibly will help the individual to prevent the establishment of infection [152]. The bacterial infection is transmitted by adolescents and adults, so the development of new vaccines is focused on vaccines intended for adolescents and adults. This vaccine is not suggested to HIV-affected individuals as it is effective in infants up to some extent. Modeling study revealed that a vaccine might aid to prevent active TB disease during the first two decades in adolescents and infants [153]. In another study, it has been found that vaccines aimed at adolescents and adults possibly improve consequence of TB burden than vaccine target at infants globally over the time 2024–2050, and such vaccines are considered to be comparatively cost-effective [154]. A vaccine must work in a way that is expected to acts totally independent of drug targets and work uniformly against both drug-sensitive and drug-resistant strains of *Mtb*. The development of vaccine faces different hurdles like lack of support from biopharmaceutical companies, economic barriers, scientific barriers, lack of predictive animal model, lack of investment in research, and development of TB. Regardless of these shortcomings, about 13 vaccines are presently being tested in clinical patients and are under global pipelines in order to treat TB infections. VPM 1002 (recombinant BCG) and MTBVAC (live-attenuated *Mtb*) are under clinical trials to prevent active TB disease in infants. Vaccae (heat-inactivated, whole-cell *Mycobacterium vaccae*), RUTI (detoxified, fragmented *Mtb*), and ID93+GLA-SE (adjuvanted recombinant protein expressing *Mtb* antigens Rv3620, Rv3619, Rv2608, and Rv1813) are under different clinical trials for prevention of active TB disease in individuals with LTBI, adjunctive immunotherapy in individuals with LTBI, and management of active TB disease reappearance in recently cured patients, respectively. H1 or H56:IC31 (adjuvanted recombinant protein expressing *Mtb* antigens), M72/ASO1E (adjuvanted recombinant protein expressing *Mtb* antigens 32A and 39A), DAR-901 (whole-cell, inactivated nontuberculous *Mycobacterium*), H4:IC31 (adjuvanted recombinant protein expressing *Mtb* antigens Ag85B and TB10.4), Ad5 Ag85A (human adenovirus 5, viral vector expressing *Mtb* antigen Ag85A), ChAdOx1-85A/MVA85A (chimp adenovirus/modified Vaccinia Virus Ankara, a viral vector heterologous prime–boost expressing *Mtb* antigen Ag85A), MVA85A/MVA85A (modified Vaccinia Virus Ankara, a viral vector intradermal followed by aerosol; prime–boost vaccine), and TB/FLU-04L (influenza A virus, viral vector) are under different phase of clinical trial for the control and prevention of TB disease in LTBI and uninfected individuals [153].

As per WHO reports, it has been revealed that about 80% of active TB patients are infected with *Mtb* strains every year. These patients are completely prone to all existing antibiotics and the rest of the patients to resistant strains (5.3% MDR and 13.3% isoniazid monoresistant) [145, 155, 156]. In 2014, around 1.9 million individuals developed drug-resistant TB, so there is an exigency of longer and efficient treatment schedules for patients with MDR-TB. Lists of drugs which are used to treat TB are represented in Table 5.1 [157–161].

WHO treatment regimen for LTBI includes 6 to 9 months treatment of isoniazid, 3 months treatment of rifapentine and isoniazid, 3 to 4 months treatment of isoniazid and rifampicin, or rifampicin alone [156]. Populations with isoniazid monoresistant strains were given a regimen containing rifampicin. It is a very effective treatment, but patient compliance can be reduced during the long-term treatment [162].

The present treatment regimen for drug-sensitive TB comprises minimum of 6 months of treatment of isoniazid, rifampicin, pyrazinamide, and ethambutol for the initial 2 months, which refers to as the early phase of treatment. It is followed by the continuation phase involving 4 months treatment of isoniazid and rifampicin. Efficacy of treatment is monitored from time to time via different TB diagnostic tests. The standard regimen has higher efficacy and high success rate [153].

The most common monitoring approach for TB is directly observed therapy (DOT), where health professional supervised each and every dose of treatment schedule. Various alternative methods regarding DOT are being attempted presently to improve observance, which include the use of call centers to follow-up with patients, smart pillboxes, and video DOT. It seems to be fundamental to utilize team-based technologies, which integrate counseling, education, and patient empowerment [163].

To minimize disease transmission and reducing drug resistance, timely diagnosis and initiation of an effectual treatment against active drug-resistant TB disease are very significant [164]. The current TB therapies for drug-resistant TB include administration of drugs like fluoroquinolones (levofloxacin, moxifloxacin, and

Table 5.1 Pharmacological overview of anti-TB drugs

S. No.	Name of drug (abbreviation)	Route	Dose regimen	Mode of action	Side effects
First-line antitubercular drugs					
1.	Isoniazid (INH)	Oral, intramuscular, or intravenous	5 mg/kg for adults, 10–20 mg/kg for children	Inhibits fatty acid synthesis via inhibition of InhA, NADH-specific enoyl-acyl carrier protein reductase	Psychosis, coma, mental confusion, convulsive seizures, and peripheral neuropathy
2.	Rifampin (RIF)	Oral or intravenous	10 mg/kg, but not exceed above 600 mg/day	Binds to β-subunit of RNA polymerase and inhibits transcription	Hepatitis, renal failure, hemolytic anemia, and thrombocytopenia
3.	Pyrazinamide (PZA)	Oral	20–25 mg/kg/day or 50–70 mg/kg thrice a week	Cellular acidification	Hepatotoxicity, severe exanthema, and acute arthritis in gouty individuals
4.	Ethambutol (ETH)	Oral	15–25 mg/kg/day	Inhibits synthesis of cell wall via acting on arabinosyl transferases	Hepatotoxicity and optic neuropathy
5.	Rifabutin (RIFAB)	Oral	300 mg/day	Binds to β-subunit of RNA polymerase and inhibits transcription	Hepatitis, diarrhea, thrombocytopenia
6.	Streptomycin (STR)	Intravenous or intramuscular	1 g/day	Binds to the conserved A region of 16S rRNA of 30s ribosomal subunit and inhibits translation	Neurotoxic reactions like peripheral neuritis, optic nerve dysfunction, cochlear and vestibular dysfunction, arachnoiditis, and encephalopathy
Second-line antituberculosis drugs (A) Fluoroquinolones					
7.	Gatifloxacin (GATI)	Oral or intravenous	400 mg/day	Inhibition of ATP-dependent enzymes topoisomerase II and IV	Dizziness, nausea, headaches, and diarrhea
8.	Levofloxacin (LEV)	Oral	500–1000 mg/day	Inhibiting ATP-dependent enzymes topoisomerase II and IV	Hepatotoxicity, joint pain, tendon rupture, phototoxicity, and prolongation of QT interval

9.	Moxifloxacin (MOXI)	Oral or intravenous	400 mg/day	Inhibiting ATP-dependent enzymes topoisomerase II and IV	Diarrhea, QT_c prolongation
10.	Ciprofloxacin (CIP)	Oral	1500 mg/day	Inhibit DNA gyrase activity	Abdominal discomfort, aerophagy, diarrhea, anorexia, tremors, and mood disorders
11.	Ofloxacin (OFL)	Oral	800 mg/day but in two divided doses	Inhibit DNA gyrase activity	Abdominal discomfort, aerophagy, diarrhea, anorexia, tremors, and mood disorders
(B) Injectable antitubercular drugs					
12.	Kanamycin (KAN)	Intravenous or intramuscular	1 g/day	Binds to the conserved A region of 16S rRNA of 30s ribosomal subunit and inhibits translation	Renal and eighth cranial-nerve impairment, intestinal obstruction
13.	Amikacin (AMI)	Intravenous or intramuscular	1 g/day	Binds to the conserved A region of 16S rRNA of 30s ribosomal subunit and inhibits translation	Eighth cranial nerve impairment leading to hearing loss, loss of balance, neurotoxicity, and nephrotoxicity
14.	Capreomycin (CAP)	Intravenous or intramuscular	1 g/day	Inhibits translation	Leukopenia, neuromuscular blockade, auditory and vestibular ototoxicity, nephrotoxicity, unusual bleeding
Other second-line antitubercular drugs					
15.	Para-aminosalicylic acid (PAS)	Oral	8–12 g/day in 2–3 different doses	Inhibits dihydrofolate reductase (DHFR) in folate pathway	Interferes with thyroid metabolism and uptake of vitamin B_{12}
16.	Ethionamide (ETA)	Oral	750 mg/day	Inhibits translation by interfering with the activity of the inhA gene of *Mtb*, thereby preventing the mycolic acid biosynthesis and affecting the cell membrane of bacteria	Metallic taste, abdominal pain, diarrhea, excessive salivation, stomatitis, anorexia

(continued)

Table 5.1 (continued)

S. No.	Name of drug (abbreviation)	Route	Dose regimen	Mode of action	Side effects
17.	Cycloserine (CYS)	Oral	500–750 mg/day	Inhibits alanine racemase (Alr, converts L-alanine to D-alanine) and D-alanine:D-alanine ligase (Ddl) which synthesizes the pentapeptide core using D-alanine, thus inhibits the formation of peptidoglycans, involved in maintenance and biosynthesis of cell wall	Neurological and psychiatric adverse effects
18.	Thiacetazone (TAC)	Oral	150 mg/day	Inhibits the reproduction of bacteria	Loss of appetite, diarrhea, skin rashes, aching joints/muscles, clumsiness, tingling/burning sensation in the hands and feet
19.	Clarithromycin (CLA)	Oral	250–1000 mg/day	Inhibits translation by binding to the 50S ribosomal subunit	Diarrhea, abdominal pain, rash
20.	Linezolid (LIN)	Oral or intravenous	600 and 400 mg in every 12 h for severe infections and uncomplicated infection, respectively	Binds to 23S rRNA and inhibits translation by interfering with proper binding of formyl-methionine tRNA	Peripheral and optic neuropathy, acidosis, diarrhea
Other antitubercular drugs					
21.	Bedaquiline (TMC-207)	Oral	400 mg/day for first 2 weeks, followed by 200 mg thrice per week for next 22 weeks	Inhibits c subunit of ATP synthase leading to inadequate synthesis of ATP	Hepatitis, diarrhea, hemoptysis, rash, somnolence, QT prolongation, arthralgia, phospholipidosis

22.	Delamanid (OPC67683)	Oral	100 mg twice/day for 24 weeks	Inhibits mycolic acid synthesis, thereby preventing the production of mycobacterial cell envelope	Insomnia, upper abdominal pain, cardiotoxicity
23.	Pretomanid (PA-824)	Oral	200 mg/day	Inhibits biosynthesis of mycolic acid, thus blocks the cell wall production	Increased liver enzymes, visual impairment, abnormal weight loss, diarrhea
24.	Sutezolid (STZ)	Oral	600 mg twice/day or 1200 mg/day	Inhibits translation	No severe adverse events reported in 14-day early bactericidal activity trial

gatifloxacin), aminoglycosides (kanamycin, amikacin, streptomycin, and capreomycin), ethionamides, oxazolidinones (cycloserine and linezolid), nicotinamide analog (pyrazinamide), isonicotinic acid hydrazide (high-dose isoniazid), amino alcohols (ethambutol), amino-phenol (para-aminosalicylic acid), diarylquinoline (bedaquiline), nitro-dihydro-imidazooxazole (delamanid), and thiosemicarbazone (thioacetazone). These treatment regimens are relatively long with reduced efficacy and high toxicity. There is a need for continuous monitoring of regular medical examination to determine toxicity-related parameters [165]. This regimen is being used by various countries because of its promising result, and these treatment guidelines were updated by WHO in May 2016 for active drug-resistant TB. Although it is likely to give assistance to the majority of patients with active MDR-TB, but resistance develops if it is taken inappropriately or without proper drug sensitivity testing [166]. Due to increase in the number of TB patients, efficient treatment regimens cannot be created or can fail. These cases of XDR-TB have been present in numerous countries such as India, China, South Africa, and Russia. In such cases, bedaquiline or delamanid treatment can be effective for these patients, although there are challenges to compose an effective treatment option. Because of limited access to these drugs, patients can remain therapeutically pitiable. Thus, there are large numbers of patients who remain incurable with drug-resistant TB and pose a major challenge for global TB control [153]. It has been evident that totally drug-resistant strains emphasize two major issues: First, the development and introduction of newly approved drugs did not take speed along with the appearance of new drug-resistant strains. Second, the introduction of these drugs is due to an elevated incidence of drug-resistant strains without considering the fundamental causes of the appearance of these strains and the risk of amplifying resistance toward anti-TB drug [167, 168]. Beyond the treatment regimen, surgery plays an important role to manage drug-resistant TB. Surgical treatment is an effective treatment for removing of affected area of the lung when treatment of drugs was not successful [153].

Change in gene expression profiles due to antibiotics suggests a better understanding of the consequence of a drug on the functioning of *Mtb* that can be analyzed by RNA sequencing to access the effect of target genes and underlying mechanism of drug resistance. The genes that promote antibiotic resistance are known as resistome [169]. *Mtb* can modulate their inherited expression to augment its growth within the host, thus contributing toward drug resistance systems. The drugs that target these resistance corridors can be used in combination with the preexisting antitubercular drugs as adjuvant therapy [170]. Therefore, inactivating resistance mechanisms [171] or efflux transporter inhibition [172] should be considered a better ideology to improve the current TB therapy. Risorine, a dose combination of rifampicin (200 mg), isoniazid (300 mg), and piperine (10 mg), with WHO approved anti-TB regimen is used for the treatment of drug-susceptible TB patients who developed gastrointestinal intolerance. This novel formulation is found to be much effective against drug-susceptible pulmonary TB using piperine as bioenhancer that has ability to inhibit the p-gp (efflux) transporters [173].

Intervening approaches are adopted for the new regimen, as the development of new drug is lengthy, costly, and uncertainty in results. These include the use of current anti-TB drugs which have not been broadly prescribed, elevated doses of existing antitubercular drugs, and "re-purposed" drugs. Re-purposed drugs are those drugs which were initially developed for other diseases but prove to be efficient against resistant TB like rifapentine [174, 175]. It has in vitro antimycobacterial activity similar to rifampicin that has fivefold higher half-life. Additionally, fluoroquinolones are a class of antibiotics that have excellent in vitro activity against *Mtb*. It has similar effect as isoniazid in the early phase of treatment of drug-sensitive TB. But later on, trials revealed that short fluoroquinolone-based regimens for the period of 4 months might not accomplish similar effect as the standard 6 months regimen [174].

The USFDA approved two drugs namely bedaquiline and delamanid for the management of pulmonary MDR-TB in adults [176]. In 2014, the European Commission authorized both the drugs. Both the drugs act via novel mechanisms. These drugs are very effective and have good "sterilizing" properties [177]. TB drug pipeline is now the largest in terms of drug development with numerous early TB drug discovery projects. This program has been supported by foundation of Bill & Melinda Gates for collaborative drug discovery in the field of TB. These include number of drugs, including CPZEN-45, TBI166, SQ609, SEQ-9, PBTZ169, TBA-7371, Q203, BTZ-043, GSK-070 which are under different preclinical and clinical phases [153].

HIV is an extreme challenge for global TB. It has been found that HIV-positive patients showed 26-fold additional possibility to develop active TB disease than HIV-negative persons. Positive individuals are at intense risk of progression of infection to active disease [178]. Antiretroviral therapy (ART) has been confirmed to decrease the incidence of active TB disease by giving immune reconstitution. To reduce severe illnesses of TB among HIV-positive individuals, the combination approach involves the use of ART and isoniazid treatment, which is an effective one. Five percent to 40% of patients with TB are at the commencing of ART in the area of sub-Saharan Africa [153, 179].

5.3.1 Drawbacks of the Current Treatment

Efforts are ongoing to control TB, as current TB treatment options are also associated with some pitfalls, which are described below.

TB remains a serious health issue in industrialized countries having specific socioeconomic factors. The main challenge is the early diagnosis of TB and its growing pattern of resistance towards drugs. The early diagnosis, identification of species, and treatment of the patient are necessary to reduce the rate of transmission of *Mtb* and for the elimination of the disease. Also, there is a high risk of developing active form of disease if a person has LTBI and, thus, requires early identification for disease control. Conventional methods for diagnosis rely on medical record of patient, TST, bacteriological examination, and chest X-rays. The TST is being used for TB diagnosis since 1910. It requires 48–72 h after administration of tuberculin. The culture filtrate of tubercle bacilli results in formation of a protein-purified derivative, which is the basis for this test. There are about 200 antigens present both in bacilli BCG and in majority of non-TB bacteria. It displays low specificity of the test and very less chances for the detection of LTBI. Error can take place during test and thus can produce false results. Booster phenomenon can cause false-positive results in subsequent TST. Also, immunocompromised patients or illness can lead to false-negative results, including active TB [180]. As far as smear microscopy is concern, *Mtb* grows slowly and specimens for TB microscopy and culture get contaminated to varying degrees through growth of unwanted normal flora. In such cases, microscopy and culturing become difficult. Also, the cell wall contains high levels of mycolic acid making it hydrophobic in nature, thus causing difficulty in staining mycobacterial cells. This results in poor sensitivity (36–43%) of conventional smear microscopy [181]. Limitations in the culture techniques and extensive research have led to advancement in diagnostic procedures. One such example is the nucleic acid amplification (NAA) tests. Test could be performed directly by taking sputum. In these tests, *Mtb* complex is identified by amplification of target nucleic acid regions in both viable and nonviable bacilli. The two available tests are the Amplifier *Mtb* Direct test and the Amplicor *Mtb* test. The specificity of the test is very high in case of positive sputum smear. However, it has very low sensitivity in the absence of *Mtb*. NAA tests require less time as compared to culture of sputum for *Mtb*. In case of patients having suspicion of latent infection of the disease, NAA tests show more accuracy than TST. In case of pulmonary TB, NAA test results must be confirmed by sputum culture, but in case of extrapulmonary TB, NAA test results have less sensitivity and specificity. Due to these limitations, culture and sputum microscopy for TB diagnosis cannot be replaced by NAA [180]. There are numerous immune-based tests developed for the improvement of procedure for TB diagnosis. Serologic tests are based on the detection of the antibody immune response towards bacteria. A specific genomic segment in *Mtb* named RD-1 is identified, where CFP-10 and the ESAT-6 are the two proteins also present. In patients having TB infection, T cell targets these proteins. On the bases of antigen-specific T-cell reaction, there is development of new methods to diagnose TB infection. After stimulation by *Mtb* antigens, T cells release IFN-γ, showing more specificity as these are absent in BCG and non-TB mycobacteria species [182–185]. There are two types of blood tests, namely the QuantiFERON-TB and T-SPOT. The QuantiFERON-TB is developed in Australia in 1980 and is based on whole blood enzyme-linked immunosorbent assay. USFDA has approved the QuantiFERON-TB, and also there is a recommendation to replace TST. The US guidelines make it compulsary for all persons who are suspected to have TB infection for testing their blood, and if the results are positive, then the person is to be considered as infected with *Mtb*. The T-SPOT test has been allowed in some of the European countries under some circumstances. According to UK guidelines, blood test should be done in case the TST is positive and in those people who are suspected for false-negative TST. Speed and simplicity are the chief advantages of these tests in comparison to microscopy. Along with this, these tests have a high sensitivity for detection of false-negative TST in persons with latent infection and have the potential to discriminate false-positive TST in persons who are BCG vaccinated. Although there are many benefits, these diagnostic tools show some drawbacks also. The two tests show marked difference in terms of sensitivity. Thus, additional studies are required for establishing the positive predictive value [180, 186].

Drop out in TB patients have been observed during the diagnosis, before initiating or commencement of treatment [187]. In case–control study for pulmonary TB treatment, factors associated with noncompliance (patients who stopped treatment for 30 days) were intended with adjusted and unadjusted odds ratio. Different factors like age, income, education, race, HIV infection, drug use, smoking, and treatment of drugs demonstrated considerable links with the dropout of TB treatment in the unadjusted analysis. Smoking, drug use, income, and drug treatment are the features allied with treatment dropout after the adjustments. However, race, age, HIV infection, and education did not show significance. Incomplete treatment and retreatment were about four times and two times higher in probability of dropping out from TB treatment, respectively. It has also been demonstrated in an earlier study that treatment dropout arises in the first 3 months of treatment. Even though it is very complicated to expect which patient is improbable to hold, there is an urgency to recognize the menace factors for noncompliance that could assist providers to recognize individuals at an elevated risk for drop out [188]. Due to treatment dropout, resistance builds up in the TB patients that have a negative impact on controlling the diseases. Treatment of TB is long, complex, and potentially lethal, and thus premature treatment discontinuation in patients is predictable. Thus, there is a need to lessen the present length of its treatment, which exceeds more than 20 weeks. Improvement in treatment regimen, that is, treatment for shorter duration, could potentially decrease the likelihood of drug resistance [189].

There are several extrinsic and intrinsic factors, viz. formulation, solubility, and absorption that determine the bioavailability of drugs [190]. The presence of proximal phenyl ring in nitroimidazoles would be accountable for limited solubility of drugs that ultimately affect its in vivo efficacy [191].

Patients are directed to take drug with food or juice to exclude the gastrointestinal-linked adverse drug reactions of antitubercular drugs. The presence of food decreases the pharmacokinetic exposure of isoniazid and rifampicin, while pyrazinamide and ethambutol were unaffected [192, 193]. Food augments the time of gastric emptying, declining the stomach motility. Dissolution and disintegration profile influences the absorption in such a way that fatty food will not have any effect on bioavailability if the release rate of formulation is less than 85% in 10 min [194].

There are numerous comorbidities associated with TB infection, such as diabetes mellitus and HIV infection [195]. Concentrations of antitubercular drugs in serum are considerably lower in HIV/TB coinfected patients. Absorption of fixed-dose combination of drugs (rifampicin, isoniazid, pyrazinamide, and ethambutol) reduced significantly in HIV patients when the CD4 cell count is below 200 cells/mm^3 [196].

The fixed-dose combination treatment regimen for 6 months has a high success rate but has several limitations. The most common side effects are mild increases in the level of liver enzymes like aspartate aminotransferase, alanine aminotransferase, and total bilirubin, which possibly lead to jaundice asymptomatically and drug-induced hepatitis [190, 197].

Uptake of standard treatment regimen leads to hematological-allied side effects. A retrospective study involves two groups of total 560 patients where Group A received fixed-dose combination for about 2 months and group B received single formulation. Symptoms like thrombocytopenia, urticaria, and leucopenia were very common in group A as compared to group B [190].

Improper use of medication might be the cause of resistance. Poor quality of drugs, high bacterial load, and administration of rifampicin once, twice, or thrice weekly in HIV patients, where CD4 cell count below 100 cells/mm^3, and intake of drugs without supervision lead to an increased risk of rifampicin resistance [190].

Rifampicin is first-line antitubercular drug. Rifampicin has property of autoinduction as it also induces CYP3A4 isoforms. Single-dose oral treatment of rifampicin for 3 weeks leads to decreased bioavailability of drug from 93% to 68% [198]. Variable oral bioavailability, autoinduction of liver enzymes, and dose-dependent side effects lead to patients drop out and consequently developing resistance [199].

The factors that affect the bioavailability of drugs include crystalline form of drug, its manufacturing process, and characteristics of excipients. All these factors contribute toward the metabolism of rifampicin into 3-formyl rifamycin SV at low pH and are assisted by isoniazid. Rifampicin is an important part of fixed-dose combination, and its low bioavailability leads to low efficacy, therapeutic failure, and build-up of drug resistance [200]. Flavonoid glycoside from *Cuminum cyminum* enhanced the plasma concentration and area under curve of rifampicin by 35% and 53%, respectively [201]. Bedaquiline, a new class of antitubercular drug metabolized by cytochrome P4503A4 (CYP3A4), is used to treat MDR-TB. Rifampicin, being strong inducer of CYP3A4, can lead to a decrease in oral pharmacokinetic exposure of bedaquiline [202]. The other drawbacks associated with current treatment regimen include consequences of quality on success rate, undeniable requisition of DOTS, a prerequisite of therapeutic drug monitoring, nonsuperiority of fixed-dose combination over single formulation, and troublesome dose adjustment [190].

5.3.2 Future Directions in Therapeutics

There are about 7000 peptides that exist in nature and have an important function in sustaining the physiology of human beings, including actions like growth factors, neurotransmitters, hormones, and ion channel ligands. These are highly selective and specifically bind to cell surface receptors like G-protein-coupled receptors or ion channels as signaling molecules and thereby, triggering intracellular response. Peptides have emerged as novel therapeutic agents and also have excellent safety, tolerability, and efficacy profiles in clinical trials. About 140 peptide-based therapeutics are presently being evaluated in clinical trials [203].

In spite of various alternate approaches have ensued to fight against TB, antitubercular therapeutic peptides are emerging as the foremost alternative due to their distinctive mechanism of action and immunomodulation properties. These peptides are synthesized naturally, which comprises of a number of amino acids, exhibiting a possible activity against *Mtb*.

There are several human immune cells that are associated with antitubercular peptides to be used as therapeutics. Cathelicidins are small cationic antimicrobial peptides that exhibit protective function against pathogens due to the presence of conserved sequences. It displays cathelin domain at N terminus and variable domain at C terminus. N-terminal domain is associated with intracellular storage of cathelicidins [204]. The peptides like hCAP18 are produced by triggered neutrophils and epithelial cells, and then secreted into extracellular environment. These undergo cleavage by proteinase-3 into LL-37, a C terminus of hCAP18 and finally taken up by the neutrophils. These exogenous addition and endogenous expression of LL-37 are responsible for inhibition of survival of pathogen within host via nicotinamide adenine dinucleotide phosphate oxidase 2-dependent process. LL-37 also activates autophagy pathways stimulated by vitamin D [205] and checks the gene expression of autophagy-related pathways like beclin-1 and atg 5 via activation of mitogen-activated protein kinase and C/EBP [206]. Defensins are antimicrobial peptide of about 35 amino acid residues which have greatly conserved sequences of cysteine domain. They display innate immune response against pathogen via a mechanism which does not require oxygen [207]. Based on the difference in their structure, these are of three subfamilies, viz. α, β, and θ defensins. Gene expression study reveals that α-defensins are upregulated in infected individual and exhibit antitubercular effect [208]. HBD-1 and HBD-2, human β-defensins have antimicrobial activity. During infection, HBD-2 relocated to phagosomes and exerts antitubercular property. Human neutrophil peptide-1 is most common member of α-defensins subfamily which affects pathogen by forming pores in cellular membrane [209, 210]. Granulysin is a glycoprotein of family saposin that acts on bacterial membrane, leading to liposomes destruction and induction of apoptosis, hence showed antitubercular activity [211].

There are also human nonimmune cells associated with antitubercular peptides. Nonimmune cells like eosinophils, hepatocytes, and keratinocytes produce antitubercular peptides to kill the pathogen. Hepcidins are peptides produced within the liver. Iron is one of the important mineral required for survival of the pathogen. Hepcidins check the survival of pathogen via binding to ferroportin (iron exporter) to regulate iron transmembrane transport. It might restrict the growth of pathogens by damaging the mycobacterial structure [212]. HCL2 is part of the helical structure of cytochrome-C oxidase subunit 3, which shows similarity with ESAT-6 antigenic protein. CFP10 complex and ESAT-6 disintegrate the structure of the cell wall and restrict its growth within host [213]. Ubiquitin-derived peptide is posttransitional modification of peptide where ubiquitin as a signal molecule is responsible for the destruction of proteasome [41]. It is present inside lysosomes and restricts the survival of pathogen. Autophagy involves the fusion of lysosomes and phagosome containing pathogen, which leads to the delivery of ubiquitin to lysosomes

[214]. Ub2 is well-known ubiquitin-derived peptide which acts on both bacterial membrane and its cytoplasm, thus exerting antimicrobial property [215].

Research works are also directed toward bacteria associated with antitubercular peptides. Bacteriocins are peptides which are produced by both Gram-positive and Gram-negative bacteria having antitubercular activity. In Gram-negative bacteria, they are categorized into small peptides (microcins) or larger proteins (colicins). In Gram-positive bacteria, bacteriocins are divided into two classes, such as lantibiotics and the nonlantibiotics, and both are thermostable. The lantibiotics are the peptides containing varied amino acid sequences with unique thioether-based ring structures. These include Nisin, thuricin CD, subtilin, and lacticin 3147. Nisin is a protein produced by *Lactococcus lactis* containing 34 amino acid sequences approved by USFDA as safe food additives. It decreased the gradient of proton motive force in bacteria and exerted an inhibitory effect on the growth of bacteria. It is found that nisin at the concentration of 2.5 mg/mL inhibits the growth of *Mycobacterium bovis* BCG [216]. Lacticin 3147 produced by *Lactococcus lactis* hinders the formation of cell wall and then binds to precursor of peptidoglycan, thus producing pores in the cell membrane of bacteria [217]. Nocardithiocin, a distinctive antibiotic produced by strain IFM 0757 of *Nocardia pseudobrasiliensis*, was active against sensitive and resistant strains with MIC of 0.025 mg/mL. The nonlantibiotics are peptides containing 25–60 amino acids, such as class-II bacteriocins produced by lactic acid bacteria [218].

Research works are undergoing for fungus-derived antitubercular peptides. Fungi are potential sources of lead bioactive compounds. There are a number of peptides that are produced by fungi with greater biotechnological potential to restrict the growth of bacteria. Calpinactam, antimycobacterial hexapeptide, produced by *Mortierella alpina* inhibits the growth of bacteria by disturbing the cell wall biosynthesis, and its MIC is found to be 12.5 mg/mL [219]. Trichoderins, aminolipopeptides, isolated from marine fungus of *Trichoderma* inhibits the growth of bacteria by encumbering the mode of ATP synthesis. They displayed antimycobacterial activity against active and dormant bacilli at the concentration of 0.02–2.0 mg/mL [220]. Bisdethiobis is a methylsulfanyl apoaranotin, a bioactive peptide produced by *Aspergillus terreus* BCC 4651 that inhibits the growth of *Mtb* H37Ra with MIC value of 1.56 mg/mL. Cordycommunin produced by fungus Ophiocordyceps communis BCC 16475 restricts the survival of Mtb H37Ra with MIC of 15 mM [221].

Research works are also directed for venom-derived antitubercular peptides. It has been revealed that reptile or arthropod venom is associated with anti-TB activity. Venom of snake is a mixture of proteins and bioactive polypeptides. Due to their divergent physiological and pharmacological effects, the proteins are of greater biological significance, thus representing an important tool for the development of drugs [222]. vgf-1 produced by *Naja atra* displays a significant activity against MDR strain with MIC of 8.5 mg/L [223]. Bhunia et al. demonstrate that venoms isolated from *Daboia russelli russelli*, *Naja naja*, *Naja kaouthia*, and *Bungarus fasciatus* also possess activity against MDR-TB strains [224]. Pandinin 2, an antimicrobial peptide isolated from scorpion, *Pandinus imperator* venom that possess proline residue at the center and forms a "kink". It is associated with pore-forming activity and thereby, attributes to its antimicrobial activity [225].

5.4 Perspective

WHO has taken promising steps toward "ending the global TB epidemic" by 2030 through setup of concrete milestones and targets. Overall progress is happening toward the set direction but speed has to be improved to achieve the goal. In this present scenario of TB treatment, it should be worth mentioning about the followings: Correct and timely diagnosis with the availability of advance techniques is required. Proper and complete treatment should be monitored/done at an affordable cost of medicines. Vaccination can be a viable option to prevent TB, but further research is needed to develop an effective vaccine for all age groups. Drug discovery/development should be directed to new chemotype that should be active against both susceptible and resistant strains and have lesser drug–drug interaction potential, minor toxicity, shorter treatment regimen, and preferably administered through oral route. Ongoing research works on peptide-based therapeutics, immunotherapeutics, and novel targeted dosage forms can open up the window for effective mitigation of TB.

References

1. Comas I, Coscolla M, Luo T, Borrell S, Holt KE, Kato-Maeda M, Parkhill J, Malla B, Berg S, Thwaites G, Yeboah-Manu D, Bothamley G, Mei J, Wei L, Bentley S, Harris SR, Niemann S, Diel R, Aseffa A, Gao Q, Young D, Gagneux S (2013) Out-of-Africa migration and Neolithic coexpansion of Mycobacterium tuberculosis with modern humans. Nat Genet 45:1176–1182
2. Ehrt S, Schnappinger D (2009) Mycobacterial survival strategies in the phagosome: defence against host stresses. Cell Microbiol 11:1170–1178
3. Briffotaux J, Liu S, Gicquel B (2019) Genome-wide transcriptional responses of mycobacterium to antibiotics. Front Microbiol 10:249. https://doi.org/10.3389/fmicb.2019.00249
4. WHO (2019) Global tuberculosis report 2019. WHO, Geneva
5. Hayman J (1984) Mycobacterium ulcerans: an infection from Jurassic time? Lancet 2:1015–1016
6. Gutierrez MC, Brisse S, Brosch R, Fabre M, Omais B, Marmiesse M, Supply P, Vincent V (2005) Ancient origin and gene mosaicism of the progenitor of Mycobacterium tuberculosis. PLoS Pathog 1:e5
7. Cave AJE (1939) The evidence for the incidence of tuberculosis in ancient Egypt. Br J Tubercul 33:142–152
8. Brown L (1941) Radiology: the story of clinical pulmonary tuberculosis. The Williams and Wilkins, Baltimore, MD
9. Daniel TM (2000) The origins and precolonial epidemiology of tuberculosis in the Americas: can we figure them out? Int J Tuberc Lung Dis 4:395–400
10. Salo WL, Aufderheide AC, Buikstra J, Holcomb TA (1994) Identification of Mycobacterium tuberculosis DNA in a pre-Columbian Peruvian mummy. Proc Natl Acad Sci U S A 91:2091–2094
11. Allison MJ, Mendoza D, Pezzia A (1973) Documentation of a case of tuberculosis in Pre-Columbian America. Am Rev Respir Dis 107:985–991

12. Glaziou P, Floyd K, Raviglione MC (2018) Global epidemiology of tuberculosis. Semin Respir Crit Care Med 39:271–285
13. Brosch R, Gordon SV, Marmiesse M, Brodin P, Buchrieser C, Eiglmeier K, Garnier T, Gutierrez C, Hewinson G, Kremer K, Parsons LM, Pym AS, Samper S, van Soolingen D, Cole ST (2002) A new evolutionary scenario for the Mycobacterium tuberculosis complex. Proc Natl Acad Sci U S A 99:3684–3689
14. Saeed BW (2006) Malignant tuberculosis. J Ayub Med Coll Abbottabad 18:1–2
15. Bloom BR, Murray CJL (1992) Tuberculosis: commentary on a reemergent killer. Science 257:1055–1064
16. Barberis I, Bragazzi NL, Galluzzo L, Martini M (2017) The history of tuberculosis: from the first historical records to the isolation of Koch's bacillus. J Prev Med Hyg 58:E9–E12
17. Gradmann C (2001) Robert Koch and the pressures of scientific research: tuberculosis and tuberculin. Med Hist 45:1–32
18. Daniel TM (2011) Hermann Brehmer and the origins of tuberculosis sanatoria. Int J Tuberc Lung Dis 15:161–162
19. Veron LJ, Blanc LJ, Suchi M, Raviglione MC (2004) DOTS expansion: will we reach the 2005 targets? Int J Tuberc Lung Dis 8:139–146
20. Maher D, Blanc L, Raviglione M (2004) WHO policies for tuberculosis control. Lancet 363:1911
21. WHO (2018) Global tuberculosis report 2018. WHO, Geneva
22. CDC (n.d.) Self-study modules on tuberculosis. Centers for Disease Control and Prevention website. http://www.cdc.gov/tb/education/ssmodules/. Updated 11 May 2016. Accessed 14 Jun 2016
23. Cole ST, Brosch R, Parkhill J, Garnier T, Churcher C, Harris D, Gordon SV, Eiglmeier K, Gas S, Barry CE III, Tekaia F, Badcock K, Basham D, Brown D, Chillingworth T, Connor R, Davies R, Devlin K, Feltwell T, Gentles S, Hamlin N, Holroyd S, Hornsby T, Jagels K, Krogh A, McLean J, Moule S, Murphy L, Oliver K, Osborne J, Quail MA, Rajandream MA, Rogers J, Rutter S, Seeger K, Skelton J, Squares R, Squares S, Sulston JE, Taylor K, Whitehead S, Barrell BG (1998) Deciphering the biology of Mycobacterium tuberculosis from the complete genome sequence. Nature 393:537–544
24. Lee RB, Li W, Chatterjee D, Lee RE (2005) Rapid structural characterization of the arabinogalactan and lipoarabinomannan in live mycobacterial cells using 2D and 3D HR-MAS NMR: structural changes in the arabinan due to ethambutol treatment and gene mutation are observed. Glycobiology 15:139–151
25. Knechel NA (2009) Tuberculosis: pathophysiology, clinical features, and diagnosis. Crit Care Nurse 29:34–43
26. CDC (2009) Interactive core curriculum on tuberculosis. Centers for Disease Control and Prevention. Available from http://www.cdc.gov/tb/webcourses/CoreCurr/TB_Course/Menu/frameset_internet.htm
27. Jensen PA, Lambert LA, Iademarco MF, Ridzon R, Centers for Disease Control and Prevention (2005) Guidelines for preventing the transmission of Mycobacterium tuberculosis in health-care settings, 2005. MMWR Recommend Rep 54:1–141
28. Frieden TR, Sterling TR, Munsiff SS, Watt CJ, Dye C (2003) Tuberculosis. Lancet 362:887–899
29. Paton NI, Chua YK, Earnest A, Chee CB (2004) Randomized controlled trial of nutritional supplementation in patients with newly diagnosed tuberculosis and wasting. Am J Clin Nutr 80:450–465
30. Ddungu H, Johnson JL, Smieja M, Mayanja-Kizza H (2006) Digital clubbing in tuberculosis—relationship to HIV infection, extent of disease and hypoalbuminemia. BMC Infect Dis 6:1–7
31. Elder NC (1992) Extrapulmonary tuberculosis. Arch Fam Med 1:91–98

32. Ehtesham SE, Grover S (2019) Mycobacterium tuberculosis: molecular infection biology, pathogenesis, diagnostics and new interventions. Springer Nature Singapore Pte Ltd., New Delhi
33. Wise GJ, Marella VK (2003) Genitourinary manifestations of tuberculosis. Urol Clin North Am 30:111–121
34. Pigrau-Serrallach C, Rodriguez-Pardo D (2013) Bone and joint tuberculosis. Eur Spine J 22: S556–S566
35. Harney M, Hone S, Timon C, Donnelly M (2000) Laryngeal tuberculosis: an important diagnosis. J Laryngol Otol 114:878–880
36. Ruiz-Manzano J, Blanquer R, Calpe JL, Caminero JA, Cayla J, Dominguez JA, Garcia JM, Vidal R (2008) Diagnosis and treatment of tuberculosis. Arch Bronconeumol 44:551–566
37. Wang JY, Hsueh PR, Wang SK, I-Shiow J, Li-Na L, Yuang-Shuang L, Pan-Chyr Y, Kwen-Tay L (2007) Disseminated tuberculosis: a 10-year experience in a medical center. Medicine 86:39–46
38. Jauregui-Amezaga A, Turon F, Ordás I, Gallego M, Feu F, Ricart E, Panés J (2013) Risk of developing tuberculosis under anti-TNF treatment despite latent infection screening. J Crohn Colit 7:208–212
39. Skinner HA (1961) The origin of medical terms, 2nd edn. The Williams and Wilkins Company, Baltimore, MD
40. Wain H (1958) The story behind the word. Charles C. Thomas, Chicago, IL
41. Purdy GE, Russell DG (2007) Lysosomal ubiquitin and the demise of Mycobacterium tuberculosis. Cell Microbiol 9:2768–2774
42. Lin PL, Ford CB, Coleman MT, Myers AJ, Gawande R, Ioerger T, Sacchettini J, Fortune SM, Flynn JL (2014) Sterilization of granulomas is common in active and latent tuberculosis despite within-host variability in bacterial killing. Nat Med 20:75–79
43. Antonelli LR, Gigliotti Rothfuchs A, Goncalves R, Roffe E, Cheever AW, Bafica A, Salazar AM, Feng CG, Sher A (2010) Intranasal poly-IC treatment exacerbates tuberculosis in mice through the pulmonary recruitment of a pathogen-permissive monocyte/macrophage population. J Clin Investig 120:1674–1682
44. Pai M, Denkinger CM, Kik SV, Rangaka MX, Zwerling A, Oxlade O, Metcalfe JZ, Cattamanchi A, Dowdy DW, Dheda K, Banaei N (2014) Gamma interferon release assays for detection of Mycobacterium tuberculosis infection. Clin Microbiol Rev 27:3–20
45. Arend SM, van Meijgaarden KE, de Boer K, de Palou EC, van Soolingen D, Ottenhoff TH, van Dissel JT (2002) Tuberculin skin testing and *in vitro* T cell responses to ESAT-6 and culture filtrate protein 10 after infection with Mycobacterium marinum or M. kansasii. J Infect Dis 186:1797–1807
46. Wang J, McIntosh F, Radomski N, Dewar K, Simeone R, Enninga J, Brosch R, Rocha EP, Veyrier FJ, Behr MA (2015) Insights on the emergence of Mycobacterium tuberculosis from the analysis of Mycobacterium kansasii. Genome Biol Evol 7:856–870
47. Marakalala MJ, Raju RM, Sharma K, Zhang YJ, Eugenin EA, Prideaux B, Daudelin IB, Chen PY, Booty MG, Kim JH, Eum SY, Via LE, Behar SM, Barry CE, Mann M, Dartois V, Rubin EJ (2016) Inflammatory signaling in human tuberculosis granulomas is spatially organized. Nat Med 22:531–538
48. Rich AR (1951) The pathogenesis of tuberculosis, 2nd edn. Charles C. Thomas, Chicago, IL
49. Zumla A, James GD (1996) Granulomatous infections: etiology and classification. Clin Infect Dis 72:146–158
50. Welin A, Raffetseder J, Eklund D, Stendahl O, Lerm M (2011) Importance of phagosomal functionality for growth restriction of Mycobacterium tuberculosis in primary human macrophages. J Innate Immun 3:508–518
51. Li W, Xie J (2011) Role of mycobacteria effectors in phagosome maturation blockage and new drug targets discovery. J Cell Biochem 112:2688–2693

52. Mishra AK, Driessen NN, Appelmelk BJ, Besra GS (2011) Lipoarabinomannan and related glycoconjugates: structure, biogenesis and role in Mycobacterium tuberculosis physiology and host–pathogen interaction. FEMS Microbiol Rev 35:1126–1157
53. Indrigo J, Hunter RL Jr, Actor JK (2003) Cord factor trehalose 6,6-dimycolate (TDM) mediates trafficking events during mycobacterial infection of murine macrophages. Microbiology 149:2049–2059
54. Camacho LR, Constant P, Raynaud C, Laneelle MA, Triccas JA, Gicquel B, Daffe M, Guilhot C (2001) Analysis of the phthiocerol dimycocerosate locus of Mycobacterium tuberculosis. Evidence that this lipid is involved in the cell wall permeability barrier. J Biol Chem 76:19845–19854
55. Kaplan MH, Armstrong D, Rosen P (1974) Tuberculosis complicating neoplastic disease: a review of 201 cases. Cancer 33:850–858
56. Ghon A (1916) The primary lung focus of tuberculosis in children [Translation by King DB]. Churchill, London
57. Salyer WR, Salyer DC, Baker RD (1974) Primary complex of cryptococcus and pulmonary lymph nodes. J Infect Dis 130:74–77
58. Hunter RL (2018) The pathogenesis of tuberculosis: the early infiltrate of post-primary (adult pulmonary) tuberculosis: a distinct disease entity. Front Immunol 9:2108
59. Scriba TJ, Penn-Nicholson A, Shankar S, Hraha T, Thompson EG, Sterling D, Nemes E, Darboe F, Suliman S, Amon LM, Mahomed H, Erasmus M, Whatney W, Johnson JL, Boom WH, Hatherill M, Valvo J, De Groote MA, Ochsner UA, Aderem A, Hanekom WA, Zak DE (2017) Sequential inflammatory processes define human progression from M. tuberculosis infection to tuberculosis disease. PLoS Pathog 13:e1006687
60. Ziemele B, Ranka R, Ozere I (2017) Pediatric and adolescent tuberculosis in Latvia, 2011-2014: case detection, diagnosis and treatment. Int J Tuberc Lung Dis 21:637–645
61. Esmail H, Lai RP, Lesosky M, Wilkinson KA, Graham CM, Coussens AK, Oni T, Warwick JM, Said-Hartley Q, Koegelenberg CF, Walzl G, Flynn JL, Young DB, Barry Iii CE, O'Garra A, Wilkinson RJ (2016) Characterization of progressive HIV-associated tuberculosis using 2-deoxy2-[18F] fluoro-D-glucose positron emission and computed tomography. Nat Med 22:1090–1093
62. Medlar EM (1955) The behavior of pulmonary tuberculosis lesion: a pathological study. Am Rev Tubercul 71:1–244
63. Sharma SK, Mohan A (2011) Tuberculosis, 2nd edn. Jaypee Brothers Medical Publishers (P) LTD, New Delhi
64. Bals R, Hiemstra PS (2004) Innate immunity in the lung: how epithelial cells fight against respiratory pathogens. Eur Respir J 23:327–333
65. Kato A, Schleimer RP (2007) Beyond inflammation: airway epithelial cells are at the interface of innate and adaptive immunity. Curr Opin Immunol 19:711–720
66. Stanke F (2015) The contribution of the airway epithelial cell to host defense. Mediators Inflamm 2015:463016
67. Kleinnijenhuis J, Oosting M, Joosten LAB, Netea MG, Van Crevel R (2011) Innate immune recognition of Mycobacterium tuberculosis. Clin Dev Immunol 2011:405310. https://doi.org/10.1155/2011/405310
68. Mayer AK, Muehmer M, Mages J, Gueinzius K, Hess C, Heeg K, Bals R, Lang R, Dalpke AH (2007) Differential recognition of TLR-dependent microbial ligands in human bronchial epithelial cells. J Immunol 178:3134–3142
69. Scordo JM, Knoell DL, Torrelles JB (2016) Alveolar epithelial cells in Mycobacterium tuberculosis infection: active players or innocent bystanders. J Innate Immun 8:3–14
70. Gomez MI, Prince A (2008) Airway epithelial cell signaling in response to bacterial pathogens. Pediatr Pulmonol 43:11–19
71. Cooper AM, Khader SA (2008) The role of cytokines in the initiation, expansion, and control of cellular immunity to tuberculosis. J Immunol 226:191–204

72. Lee HM, Shin DM, Jo EK (2009) Mycobacterium tuberculosis induces the production of tumor necrosis factor-α, interleukin-6, and CXCL8 in pulmonary epithelial cells through reactive oxygen species-dependent mitogen-activated protein kinase activation. J Bacteriol Virol 39:1–10
73. Lin Y, Zhang M, Barnes PF (1998) Chemokine production by a human alveolar epithelial cell line in response to Mycobacterium tuberculosis. Infect Immun 66:1121–1126
74. Nakanaga T, Nadel JA, Ueki IF, Koff JL, Shao MX (2007) Regulation of interleukin-8 via an airway epithelial signaling cascade. Am J Physiol Lung Cell Mol Physiol 292:1289–1296
75. Sharma M, Sharma S, Roy S, Varma S, Bose M (2007) Pulmonary epithelial cells are a source of interferon-gamma in response to Mycobacterium tuberculosis infection. Immunol Cell Biol 85:229–237
76. Peters W, Ernst JD (2003) Mechanisms of cell recruitment in the immune response to Mycobacterium tuberculosis. Microbes Infect 5:151–158
77. Harriff MJ, Cansler ME, Toren KG, Canfield ET, Kwak S, Gold MC, Lewinsohn DM (2014) Human lung epithelial cells contain Mycobacterium tuberculosis in a late endosomal vacuole and are efficiently recognized by CD8+ T cells. PLoS One 9:e97515
78. Gupta N, Kumar R, Agrawal B (2018) New players in immunity to tuberculosis: the host microbiome, lung epithelium, and innate immune cells. Front Immunol 9:709. https://doi.org/10.3389/fimmu.2018.0070
79. Lasco TM, Turner OC, Cassone L, Sugawara I, Yamada H, McMurray DN, Orme LM (2004) Rapid accumulation of eosinophils in lung lesions in guinea pigs infected with Mycobacterium tuberculosis. Infect Immun 2:1147–1149
80. Appelberg R (2007) Neutrophils and intracellular pathogens: beyond phagocytosis and killing. Trends Microbiol 2:87–92
81. Topham NJ, Hewitt EW (2009) Natural killer cell cytotoxicity: how do they pull the trigger? Immunology 1:7–15
82. Yoon SR, Kim T-D, Choi I (2015) Understanding of molecular mechanisms in natural killer cell therapy. Exp Mol Med 2:e141
83. Cheent K, Khakoo SI (2009) Natural killer cells: integrating diversity with function. Immunology 4:449–457
84. Esin S, Batoni G, Counoupas C, Stringaro A, Brancatisano FL, Colone M, Maisetta G, Florio W, Arancia G, Campa M (2008) Direct binding of human NK cell natural cytotoxicity receptor NKp44 to the surfaces of mycobacteria and other bacteria. Infect Immun 4:1719–1727
85. Guerra C, Johal K, Morris D, Moreno S, Alvarado O, Gray D, Tanzil M, Pearce D, Venketaraman V (2012) Control of Mycobacterium tuberculosis growth by activated natural killer cells. Clin Exp Immunol 1:142–152
86. Roy S, Barnes P, Garg A, Wu S, Cosman D, Vankayalapati R (2008) NK cells lyse T regulatory cells that expand in response to an intracellular pathogen. J Immunol 1:1729–1736
87. Kulprannet M, Sukwit S, Sumransuro K, Chuenchitra T (2007) Cytokine production in NK and NKT cells from Mycobacterium tuberculosis infected patients. Southeast Asian J Trop Med Public Health 2:370–375
88. Bozzano F, Costa P, Passalacqua G, Dodi F, Ravera S, Pagano G, Canonica GW, Moretta L, De Maria A (2009) Functionally relevant decreases in activatory receptor expression on NK cells are associated with pulmonary tuberculosis in vivo and persist after successful treatment. Int Immunol 7:779–791
89. Marcenaro E, Ferranti B, Falco M, Moretta L, Moretta A (2008) Human NK cells directly recognize Mycobacterium bovis via TLR2 and acquire the ability to kill monocyte-derived DC. Int Immunol 9:1155–1167
90. Kumar V, Delovitch TL (2014) Different subsets of natural killer T cells may vary in their roles in health and disease. Immunology 3:321–336
91. Brennan P, Brigl M, Brenner M (2013) Invariant natural killer T cells: an innate activation scheme linked to diverse effector functions. Nat Rev Immunol 2:101–117

92. Sada-Ovalle I, Chiba A, Gonzales A, Brenner MB, Behar SM (2008) Innate invariant NKT cells recognize Mycobacterium tuberculosis–infected macrophages, produce interferon-γ, and kill intracellular bacteria. PLoS Pathog 12:e1000239
93. Kee SJ, Kwon YS, Park YW, Cho YN, Lee SJ, Kim TJ, Lee SS, Jang HC, Shin MG, Shin JH, Suh SP, Ryang DW (2012) Dysfunction of natural killer T cells in patients with active Mycobacterium tuberculosis infection. Infect Immun 80:2100–2108
94. Wu C, Li Z, Fu X, Yu S, Lao S, Yang B (2015) Antigen-specific human NKT cells from tuberculosis patients produce IL-21 to help B cells for the production of immunoglobulins. Oncotarget 30:28633–28645
95. Li Z, Yang B, Zhang Y, Ma J, Chen X, Lao S, Li B, Wu C (2014) Mycobacterium tuberculosis-specific memory NKT cells in patients with tuberculous pleurisy. J Clin Immunol 8:979–990
96. Liu H, Komai-Koma M, Xu D, Liew FY (2006) Toll-like receptor 2 signaling modulates the functions of CD4+CD25+ regulatory T cells. Proc Natl Acad Sci U S A 103:7048–7053
97. Shen Y, Zhou D, Qiu L, Lai X, Simon M, Shen L, Kou Z, Wang Q, Jiang L, Estep J, Hunt R, Clagett M, Sehgal PK, Li Y, Zeng X, Morita CT, Brenner MB, Letvin NL, Chen ZW (2002) Adaptive immune response of Vγ2Vδ2+ T cells during mycobacterial infection. Science 5563:2255–2258
98. Dieli F, Ivanyi J, Marsh P, Williams A, Naylor I, Sireci G, Caccamo N, Di Sano C, Salerno A (2003) Characterization of lung γδ T cells following intranasal infection with Mycobacterium bovis bacillus Calmette-Guérin. J Immunol 1:463–469
99. Gold MC, Napier RJ, Lewinsohn DM (2015) MR1-restricted mucosal associated invariant T (MAIT) cells in the immune response to Mycobacterium tuberculosis. Immunol Rev 264:154–166
100. Howson LJ, Salio M, Cerundolo V (2015) MR1-restricted mucosal-associated invariant T cells and their activation during infectious diseases. Front Immunol 6:303
101. Chua WJ, Truscott SM, Eickhoff CS, Blazevic A, Hoft DF, Hansen TH (2012) Polyclonal mucosa-associated invariant T cells have unique innate functions in bacterial infection. Infect Immun 80:3256–3267
102. Jiang J, Yang B, An H, Wang X, Liu Y, Cao Z, Zhai F, Wang R, Cao Y, Cheng X (2016) Mucosal-associated invariant T cells from patients with tuberculosis exhibit impaired immune response. J Infect 3:338–352
103. Cella M, Miller H, Song C (2014) Beyond NK cells: the expanding universe of innate lymphoid cells. Front Immunol 5:282
104. Spits H, Cupedo T (2012) Innate lymphoid cells: emerging insights in development, lineage relationships, and function. Annu Rev Immunol 30:647–675
105. Wellmann A (2015) The modulation of innate lymphoid cells in tuberculosis and HIV co-infection. Paper presented at TB and Co-morbidities. Keystone Symposium on Host Response in Tuberculosis. Santa Fe, NM, USA
106. Randall PJ, Hsu NJ, Quesniaux V, Ryffel B, Jacobs M (2015) Mycobacterium tuberculosis infection of the 'Non-classical immune cell'. Immunol Cell Biol 93:789. https://doi.org/10.1038/icb.2015.43
107. Raad I, Hachem R, Leeds N, Sawaya R, Salem Z, Atweh S (1996) Use of adjunctive treatment with interferon-gamma in an immunocompromised patient who had refractory multidrug-resistant tuberculosis of the brain. Clin Infect Dis 22:572–574
108. Johnson JL, Nunn AJ, Fourie PB, Ormerod LP, Mugerwa RD, Mwinga A, Chintu C, Ngwira B, Onyebujoh P, Zumla A (2004) Effect of Mycobacterium vaccae (SRL172) immunotherapy on radiographic healing in tuberculosis. Int J Tuberc Lung Dis 8:1348–1354
109. Strieter RM, Remick DG, Ward PA, Spengler RN, Lynch JP, Larrick J, Kunkel SL (1988) Cellular and molecular regulation of tumor necrosis factor-alpha production by pentoxifylline. Biochem Biochem Biophys Res Commun 155:1230–1236

110. Bosho HI, Myers TG, Copp BR, McNeil MR, Wilson MA, Barry CE (2004) The transcriptional responses of Mycobacterium tuberculosis to inhibitors of metabolism: novel insights into drug mechanisms of action. J Biol Chem 279:40174–40184
111. Waddell SJ, Stabler RA, Laing K, Kremer L, Reynolds RC, Besra GS (2004) The use of microarray analysis to determine the gene expression profiles of *Mycobacterium tuberculosis* in response to anti-bacterial compounds. Tuberculosis 84:263–274
112. Manjunatha U, Boshoff HI, Barry CE (2009) The mechanism of action of PA-824: novel insights from transcriptional profiling. Communicat Integrat Biol 2:215–218
113. Liang J, Zeng F, Guo A, Liu L, Guo N, Li L, Jin J, Wu X, Liu M, Zhao D, Li Y, Jin Q, Yu L *(2011)* Microarray analysis of the chelerythrine-induced transcriptome of *Mycobacterium tuberculosis*. Curr Microbiol 62:1200–1208
114. Lee YV, Wahab HA, Choong YS (2015) Potential inhibitors for isocitrate lyase of *Mycobacterium tuberculosis* and non-*M. tuberculosis*: a summary. Biomed Res Int 2015:20
115. Fu LM, Shinnick YM (2007) Genome-wide exploration of the drug action of capreomycin on Mycobacterium tuberculosis using Affymetrix oligonucleotide GeneChips. J Infect 54:277–284
116. Lee M, Lee J, Carroll MW, Choi H, Min S, Song T, Via LE, Goldfeder LC, Kang E, Jin B, Park H, Kwak H, Kim H, Jeon HS, Jeong I, Joh JS, Chen RY, Olivier KN, Shaw PA, Follmann D, Song SD, Lee JK, Lee D, Kim CT, Dartois V, Park SK, Cho SN, Barry CE (2012) Linezolid for treatment of chronic extensively drug-resistant tuberculosis. N Engl J Med 367:1508–1518
117. Liang J, Tang X, Guo N, Zhang K, Guo A, Wu X, Wang X, Guan Z, Liu L, Shen F, Xing M, Liu L, Li L, Yu L (2012) Genome-wide expression profiling of the response to linezolid in *Mycobacterium tuberculosis*. Curr Microbiol 64:530–538
118. Habib Z, Xu W, Jamal M, Rehman K, Chen X, Dai J, Fu ZF, Chen X, Cao G (2017) Adaptive gene profiling of *Mycobacterium tuberculosis* during sub-lethal kanamycin exposure. Microb Pathog 112:243–253
119. Fishbein S, van Wyk N, Warren RM, Sampson SL (2015) Phylogeny to function: PE/PPE protein evolution and impact on Mycobacterium tuberculosis pathogenicity. Mol Microbiol 96:901–916
120. Sivaramakrishnan S, de Montellano PR (2013) The DosS-DosT/DosR mycobacterial sensor system. Biosensing 3:259–282
121. Provvedi R, Boldrin F, Falciani F, Palu G, Manganelli R (2009) Global transcriptional response to vancomycin in Mycobacterium tuberculosis. Microbiology 155:1093–1102
122. Drumm JE, Mi K, Bilder P, Sun M, Lim J, Bielefeldt-Ohmann H, Basaraba R, So M, Zhu G, Tufariello JM, Izzo AA, Orme IM, Almo SC, Leyh TS, Chan J (2009) Mycobacterium tuberculosis universal stress protein Rv2623 regulates bacillary growth by ATP-binding: requirement for establishing chronic persistent infection. PLoS Pathog 5:e1000460
123. Soetaert K, Rens C, Wang XM, De Bruyn J, Laneelle MA, Laval F, Lemassu A, Daffe M, Bifani P, Fontaine V, Philippe L (2015) Increased vancomycin susceptibility in mycobacteria: a new approach to identify synergistic activity against multidrug-resistant mycobacteria. Antimicrob Agents Chemother 59:5057–5060
124. Morris RP, Nguyen L, Gatfield J, Visconti K, Nguyen K, Schnappinger D, Ehrt S, Liu Y, Heifets L, Pieters J, Schoolnik G, Thompson CJ (2005) Ancestral antibiotic resistance in *Mycobacterium tuberculosis*. Proc Natl Acad Sci U S A 102:12200–12205
125. Geiman DE, Raghunand TR, Agarwal N, Bishai WR (2006) Differential gene expression in response to exposure to antimycobacterial agents and other stress conditions among seven Mycobacterium tuberculosis whiB-like genes. Antimicrob Agents Chemother 50:2836–2841
126. Flores AR, Parsons LM, Pavelka MSJ (2005) Genetic analysis of the beta-lactamases of Mycobacterium tuberculosis and Mycobacterium smegmatis and susceptibility to beta-lactam antibiotics. Microbiology 151:521–532
127. Espositoa S, Bianchinia S, Blasib F (2015) Bedaquiline and delamanid in tuberculosis. Expert Opin Pharmacother 16:2319–2330

128. Andries K, Verhasselt P, Guillemont J, Gohlmann HW, Neefs JM, Winkler H, Van Gestel J, Timmerman P, Zhu M, Lee E, Williams P, de Chaffoy D, Huitric E, Hoffner S, Cambau E, Truffot-Pernot C, Lounis N, Jarlier V (2005) A diarylquinoline drug active on the ATP synthase of Mycobacterium tuberculosis. Science 307:223–227
129. Koul A, Vranckx L, Dhar N, Göhlmann HW, Özdemir E, Neefs JM, Schulz M, Lu P, Mørtz E, McKinney JD, Andries K, Bald D (2014) Delayed bactericidal response of *Mycobacterium tuberculosis* to bedaquiline involves remodelling of bacterial metabolism. Nat Commun 5:3369
130. Peterson EJR, Ma S, Sherman DR, Baliga NS (2016) Network analysis identifies Rv0324 and Rv0880 as regulators of bedaquiline tolerance in *Mycobacterium tuberculosis. Nat Microbiol* 1:16078
131. Foo CS, Lupien A, Kienle M, Vocat A, Benjak A, Sommer R, Lamprecht DA, Steyn AJC, Pethe K, Piton J, Altmann KH, Cole ST (2018) Arylvinylpiperazine amides, a new class of potent inhibitors targeting QcrB of Mycobacterium tuberculosis. MBio 9:e01276-18
132. Penuelas-Urquides K, Gonzalez-Escalante L, Villarreal-Trevino L, Silva-Ramirez B, Gutierrez-Fuentes DJ, Mojica-Espinosa R, Rangel-Escareno C, Uribe-Figueroa L, Molina-Salinas GM, Davila-Velderrain J, Castorena-Torres F, Bermudez de Leon M, Said-Fernandez S (2013) Comparison of gene expression profiles between pansensitive and multidrug-resistant strains of *Mycobacterium tuberculosis.* Curr Microbiol 67:362–371
133. Yu G, Cui Z, Sun X, Peng J, Jiang J, Wu W, Huang W, Chu K, Zhang L, Ge B, Li Y (2015) Gene expression analysis of two extensively drug-resistant tuberculosis isolates show that two-component response systems enhance drug resistance. Tuberculosis 95:303–314
134. Gonzalez-Escalante L, Penuelas-Urquides K, Said-Fernandez S, Silva-Ramirez B, Bermudez De Leon M (2015) Differential expression of putative drug resistance genes in *Mycobacterium tuberculosis* clinical isolates. FEMS Microbiol Lett 362:fnv194
135. Chatterjee A, Saranath D, Bhatter P, Mistry N (2013) Global transcriptional profiling of longitudinal clinical isolates of Mycobacterium tuberculosis exhibiting rapid accumulation of drug resistance. PLoS One 8:e54717
136. De Welzen L, Eldholm V, Maharaj K, Manson AL, Earl AM, Pym AS (2017) Whole-transcriptome and genome analysis of extensively drug resistant Mycobacterium tuberculosis clinical isolates identifies downregulation of ethA as a mechanism of ethionamide resistance. Antimicrob Agents Chemother 61:e01461–e01417
137. Nebenzahl-Guimaraes H, Jacobson KR, Farhat MR, Murray MB (2014) Systematic review of allelic exchange experiments aimed at identifying mutations that confer drug resistance in Mycobacterium tuberculosis. J Antimicrob Chemother 69:331–342
138. Salamon H, Yamaguchi KD, Cirillo DM, Miotto P, Schito M, Posey J, Starks AM, Niemann S, Alland D, Hanna D, Aviles E, Perkins MD, Dolinger DL (2015) Integration of published information into a resistance-associated mutation database for Mycobacterium tuberculosis. J Infect Dis 211:S50–S57
139. Pankhurst LJ, Del Ojo Elias C, Votintseva AA, Walker TM, Cole K, Davies J, Fermont JM, Gascoyne-Binzi DM, Kohl TA, Kong C, Lemaitre N, Niemann S, Paul J, Rogers TR, Roycroft E, Smith EG, Supply P, Tang P, Wilcox MH, Wordsworth S, Wyllie D, Xu L, Crook DW (2016) Rapid, comprehensive, and affordable mycobacterial diagnosis with whole-genome sequencing: a prospective study. Lancet Respir Med 4:49–58
140. Walker TM, Kohl TA, Omar SV, Hedge J, Del Ojo Elias C, Bradley P, Iqbal Z, Feuerriegel S, Niehaus KE, Wilson DJ, Clifton DA, Kapatai G, Ip CLC, Bowden R, Drobniewski FA, Allix-Béguec C, Gaudin C, Parkhill J, Diel R, Supply P, Crook DW, Smith EG, Walker AS, Ismail N, Niemann S, Peto TEA (2015) Whole-genome sequencing for prediction of Mycobacterium tuberculosis drug susceptibility and resistance: a retrospective cohort study. Lancet Infect Dis 15:1193–1202
141. Bradley P, Gordon NC, Walker TM, Dunn L, Heys S, Huang B, Earle S, Pankhurst LJ, Anson L, de Cesare M, Piazza P, Votintseva AA, Golubchik T, Wilson DJ, Wyllie DH, Diel R, Niemann S, Feuerriegel S, Kohl TA, Ismail N, Omar SV, Smith EG, Buck D, McVean G,

Walker AS, Peto TE, Crook DW, Iqbal Z (2015) Rapid antibiotic-resistance predictions from genome sequence data for Staphylococcus aureus and Mycobacterium tuberculosis. Nat Commun 6:10063

142. Dominguez J, Boettger EC, Cirillo D, Cobelens F, Eisenach KD, Gagneux S, Hillemann D, Horsburgh R, Molina-Moya B, Niemann S, Tortoli E, Whitelaw A, Lange C (2016) Clinical implications of molecular drug resistance testing for Mycobacterium tuberculosis: a TBNET/RESIST-TB consensus statement. Int J Tuberc Lung Dis 20:24–42
143. Fine PE, Carneiro IA, Milstien JB, Clements CJ (1999) Issues relating to the use of BCG in immunization programs: a discussion document. Department of Vaccines and Biologicals, World Health Organization, Geneva
144. Luca S, Mihaescu T (2013) History of BCG vaccine. J Clin Med 8:53–58
145. WHO (2014) Guidance for national tuberculosis programmes on the management of tuberculosis in children. Available from http://apps.who.int/iris/bitstream/10665/112360/1/9789241548748_eng.pdf. Accessed Jun 2017
146. Mangtani P, Abubakar I, Ariti C, Beynon R, Pimpin L, Fine PE, Rodrigues LC, Smith PG, Lipman M, Whiting PF, Sterne JA (2014) Protection by BCG vaccine against tuberculosis: a systematic review of randomized controlled trials. Clin Infect Dis 58:470–480
147. Roy A, Eisenhut M, Harris RJ, Rodrigues LC, Sridhar S, Habermann S, Snell L, Mangtani P, Adetifa I, Lalvani A, Abubakar I (2014) Effect of BCG vaccination against Mycobacterium tuberculosis infection in children: systematic review and meta-analysis. Br Med J 349:g4643
148. Trunz BB, Fine P, Dye C (2006) Effect of BCG vaccination on childhood tuberculous meningitis and miliary tuberculosis worldwide: a meta-analysis and assessment of cost-effectiveness. Lancet 367:1173–1180
149. Barreto ML, Pereiraa SM, Pilger D, Cruzc AA, Cunha SS, Sant'Annae C, Ichiharaa MY, Genser B, Rodrigues LC (2011) Evidence of an effect of BCG revaccination on incidence of tuberculosis in school-aged children in Brazil: second report of the BCG-REVAC cluster-randomised trial. Vaccine 29:4875–4877
150. Abubakar I, Pimpin L, Ariti C, Beynon R, Mangtani P, Sterne JA, Fine PE, Smith PG, Lipman M, Elliman D, Watson JM, Drumright LN, Whiting PF, Vynnycky E, Rodrigues LC (2013) Systematic review and meta-analysis of the current evidence on the duration of protection by Bacillus Calmette–Guerin vaccination against tuberculosis. Health Technol Assess 17:1–372
151. Zwerling A, Behr MA, Verma A, Brewer TF, Menzies D, Pai M (2011) The BCG World Atlas: a database of global BCG vaccination policies and practices. PLoS Med 8:e1001012
152. Ellis RD, Hatherill M, Tait D, Snowden M, Churchyard G, Hanekom W, Evans T, Ginsberg AM (2015) Innovative clinical trial designs to rationalize TB vaccine development. Tuberculosis 95:352–357
153. Pai M, Behr MA, Dowdy DW, Dheda K, Divangahi M, Boehme CC, Ginsberg A, Swaminathan S, Spigelman S, Getahun H, Menzies D, Raviglione M (2016) Tuberculosis. Nat Rev Dis Primers 2:1–23
154. Knight GM, Griffiths UK, Sumner T, Laurence YV, Gheorghe A, Vassall A, Glaziou P, White RG (2014) Impact and cost-effectiveness of new tuberculosis vaccines in low- and middle-income countries. Proceedings of the National Academy of Sciences of the United States of America. J Infect Dis 111:15520–15525
155. WHO (2015) Global tuberculosis report 2015. WHO, Geneva
156. World Health Organization (2014) Guidelines on the management of latent tuberculosis infection. WHO, Geneva
157. Keam SJ (2019) Pretomanid: first approval. Drugs 79:1797–1803
158. Arbex MA, Varella MD, Siqueira HR, Mello FA (2010) Antituberculosis drugs: drug interactions, adverse effects, and use in special situations. Part 2: Second-line drugs. J Bras Pneumol 36:641–656
159. Lincoln EM, Sewell BH (1963) Tuberculosis in children. McGraw-Hill, New York, NY, pp 19–83

160. Semete B, Kalombo L, Katata L, Chelule P, Booysen L, Lemmer Y, Naidoo S, Ramalapa B, Hayeshi R, Swai HS (2012) Potential of improving the treatment of tuberculosis through nanomedicine. Mol Cryst Liq Cryst 556:317–330
161. Furin J, Cox H, Pai M (2019) Tuberculosis. Lancet 393:1642–1656
162. Landry J, Menzies D (2008) Preventive chemotherapy. Where has it got us? Where to go next? Int J Tuberc Lung Dis 12:1352–1364
163. Volmink J, Garner P (2007) Directly observed therapy for treating tuberculosis. Cochrane Database Syst Rev 4:CD003343
164. Dheda K, Barry CE, Maartens G (2016) Tuberculosis. Lancet 387:1211–1126
165. Calligaro GL, Moodley L, Symons G, Dheda K (2014) The medical and surgical treatment of drug-resistant tuberculosis. J Thorac Dis 6:186–195
166. World Health Organization (2016) The shorter MDR-TB regimen. WHO, Geneva. Available from http://www.who.int/tb/Short_MDR_ regimen_factsheet.pdf
167. Udwadia ZF, Amale RA, Ajbani KK, Rodrigues C (2012) Totally drug resistant tuberculosis in India. Clin Infect Dis 54:579–581
168. Udwadia ZF (2012) MDR, XDR, TDR tuberculosis: ominous progression. Thorax 67:286–288
169. Wright GD (2007) The antibiotic resistome: the nexus of chemical and genetic diversity. Nat Rev Microbiol 5:175–186
170. Jensen PA, Zhu Z, Van-Opijnen T (2017) Antibiotics disrupt coordination between transcriptional and phenotypic stress responses in pathogenic bacteria. Cell Rep 20:1705–1716
171. Wright GD (2016) Antibiotic adjuvants: rescuing antibiotics from resistance. Trends Microbiol 24:928
172. Pule CM, Sampson SL, Warren RM, Black PA, van Helden PD, Victor TC, Louw GE (2016) Efflux pump inhibitors: targeting mycobacterial efflux systems to enhance TB therapy. J Antimicrob Chemother 71:17–26
173. Vora A, Patel S, Patel K (2016) Role of risorine in the treatment of drug - susceptible pulmonary tuberculosis: a pilot study. J Assoc Physicians India 64:20–24
174. Dorman SE, Johnson JL, Goldberg S, Muzanye G, Padayatchi N, Bozeman L, Heilig CM, Bernardo J, Choudhri S, Grosset JH, Guy E, Guyadeen P, Leus MC, Maltas G, Menzies D, Nuermberger EL, Villarino M, Vernon A, Chaisson RE (2009) Substitution of moxifloxacin for isoniazid during intensive phase treatment of pulmonary tuberculosis. Am J Respir Crit Care Med 180:273–280
175. Jindani A, Harrison TS, Nunn AJ, Phillips PP, Churchyard GJ, Charalambous S, Hatherill M, Geldenhuys H, McIlleron HM, Zvada SP, Jindani A, Harrison TS, Nunn AJ, Phillips PP, Churchyard GJ, Charalambous S, Hatherill M, Geldenhuys H, McIlleron HM, Zvada SP (2014) High-dose rifapentine with moxifloxacin for pulmonary tuberculosis. N Engl J Med 371:1599–1608
176. Cox E, Laessig K (2014) FDA approval of bedaquiline — the benefit–risk balance for drug-resistant tuberculosis. N Engl J Med 371:689–691
177. Matsumoto M, Hashizume H, Tomishige T, Kawasaki M, Tsubouchi H, Sasaki H, Shimokawa Y, Komatsu M (2006) OPC-67683, a nitro-dihydroimidazooxazole derivative with promising action against tuberculosis in vitro and in mice. PLoS Med 3:e466
178. Suthar AB, Lawn SD, del Amo J, Getahun H, Dye C, Sculier D, Sterling TR, Chaisson RE, Williams BG, Harries AD, Granich RM (2012) Antiretroviral therapy for prevention of tuberculosis in adults with HIV: a systematic review and meta-analysis. PLoS Med 9: e1001270
179. Lawn SD, Harries AD, Meintjes G, Getahun H, Havlir DV, Wood R (2012) Reducing deaths from tuberculosis in antiretroviral treatment programmes in sub-Saharan Africa. AIDS 26:2121–2133
180. Tsara V, Serasli E, Christaki P (2009) Problems in diagnosis and treatment of tuberculosis infection. Hippokratia 13:20–22

181. Nema V (2012) Tuberculosis diagnostics: challenges and opportunities. Lung India 29:259–266
182. Lalvani A (2007) Diagnosing tuberculosis infection in the 21st century. Chest 131:1898–1906
183. Richeldi L (2006) An update on the diagnosis of tuberculosis infection. Am J Respir Crit Care Med 174:736–742
184. Nahid P, Pai M, Hopewell P (2006) Advances in the diagnosis and treatment of tuberculosis. Proc Am Thorac Soc 3:103–110
185. Dinnes J, Deeks J, Kunst H, Gibson A, Cummins E, Waugh N, Drobniewski F, Lalvani A (2007) A systematic review of rapid diagnostic tests for the detection of tuberculosis infection. Health Technol Assess 11:1–196
186. Menzies D, Pai M, Comstock G (2007) Meta-analysis: new test for the diagnosis of latent tuberculosis infection: areas of uncertainty and recommendations for research. Ann Intern Med 146:340–356
187. Pherson PM, Houben RMGJ, Glynn JR, Corbettc EL, Kranzer K (2014) Pre-treatment loss to follow-up in tuberculosis patients in low- and lower-middle-income countries and high-burden countries: a systematic review and meta-analysis. Bull World Health Organ 92:126. Article ID: BLT.13.124800
188. Oliveira SM, Altmayer S, Zanon M, Sidney-Filho LA, Moreira ALS, Dalcin PT, Garcez A, Hochhegger B, Moreira JS, Watte G (2018) Predictors of noncompliance to pulmonary tuberculosis treatment: an insight from South America. PLoS One 13:e0202593
189. Babiarz KS, Suen S, Goldhaber-Fiebert JD (2014) Tuberculosis treatment discontinuation and symptom persistence: an observational study of Bihar, India's public care system covering >100,000,000 inhabitants. BMC Public Health 14:418
190. Iftikhar S, Sarwar MR (2017) Potential disadvantages associated with treatment of active tuberculosis using fixed-dose combination: a review of literature. J Bas Clin Pharm 8:S131–S136
191. Mukherjee T, Boshoff H (2011) Nitroimidazoles for the treatment of TB: past, present and future. Future Med Chem 3:1427–1454
192. Requena-Méndez A (2012) Pharmacokinetics of rifampin in Peruvian tuberculosis patients with and without comorbid diabetes or HIV. Antimicrob Agents Chemother 56:2357–2363
193. Tostmann A (2013) Pharmacokinetics of first-line tuberculosis drugs in Tanzanian patients. Antimicrob Agents Chemother 57:3208–3213
194. Panchagnula R (2003) In vitro evaluation of food effect on the bioavailability of rifampicin from antituberculosis fixed dose combination formulations. Farmacoterapia 58:1099–1103
195. Hawn TR (2014) Tuberculosis vaccines and prevention of infection. Microbiol Mol Biol Rev 78:650–671
196. Suryanto A (2008) Is there an increased risk of TB relapse in patients treated with fixed-dose combination drugs in Indonesia? Int J Tuberc Lung Dis 12:174–179
197. Saukkonen JJ, Cohn DL, Jasmer RM, Schenker S, Jereb JA, Nolan CM, Peloquin CA, Gordin FM, Nunes D, Strader DB, Bernardo J, Venkataramanan R (2006) An official ATS statement: hepatotoxicity of antituberculosis therapy. Am J Respir Crit Care Med 174:935–952
198. Sutrisna EM (2015) Autoinduction properties of rifampicin on javanese tuberculosis with variant type cyp3a4∗1g. Asian J Pharm Clin Res 8:21–23
199. Sharma A, Magotra A, Bhatt S, Dogra A, Wazir P, Satti NK, Singh G, Bhusari SS, Nandi U (2018) Potential herb-drug interaction of a flavone glycoside from *Cuminum cyminum*: possible pathway for bioenhancement of rifampicin. Ind J Trad Knowl 17:776–782
200. Du Toit LC, Pillay V, Danckwerts MP (2006) Tuberculosis chemotherapy: current drug delivery approaches. Respir Res 7:118
201. Sachin BS, Sharma SC, Sethi S, Tasduq SA, Tikoo MK, Tikoo AK, Satti NK, Gupta BD, Suri KA, Johri RK, Qazi GN (2007) Herbal modulation of drug bioavailability: enhancement of rifampicin levels in plasma by herbal products and a flavonoid glycoside derived from Cuminum cyminum. Phytother Res 21:157–163

202. Svensson EM, Murray S, Karlsson MO, Dooley KE (2015) Rifampicin and rifapentine significantly reduce concentrations of bedaquiline, a new anti-TB drug. J Antimicrob Chemother 70:1106–1114
203. Fosgerau K, Hoffmann T (2015) Peptide therapeutics: current status and future directions. Drug Discov Today 20:122–128
204. Zanetti M (2004) Cathelicidins, multifunctional peptides of the innate immunity. J Leukoc Biol 75:39–48
205. Yang CS, Shin DM, Kim KH, Lee ZW, Lee CH, Park SG, Bae YS, Jo EK (2009) NADPH oxidase 2 interaction with TLR2 is required for efficient innate immune responses to mycobacteria via cathelicidin expression. J Immunol 182:3696–3705
206. Yuk JM, Shin DM, Lee HM, Yang CS, Jin HS, Kim KK, Lee ZW, Lee SH, Kim JM, Jo EK (2009) Vitamin D3 induces autophagy in human monocytes/macrophages via cathelicidin. Cell Host Microbe 6:231–243
207. Liu PT, Modlin RL (2008) Human macrophage host defense against Mycobacterium tuberculosis. Curr Opin Immunol 20:371–376
208. Jacobsen M, Repsilber D, Gutschmidt A, Neher A, Feldmann K, Mollenkopf HJ, Ziegler A, Kaufmann SH (2007) Candidate biomarkers for discrimination between infection and disease caused by Mycobacterium tuberculosis. J Mol Med 85:613–662
209. Gutierrez MG, Master SS, Singh SB, Taylor GA, Colombo MI, Deretic V (2004) Autophagy is a defense mechanism inhibiting BCG and Mycobacterium tuberculosis survival in infected macrophages. Cell 119:753–766
210. Zhu LM, Liu CH, Chen P, Dai AG, Li CX, Xiao K (2011) Multidrug-resistant tuberculosis is associated with low plasma concentrations of human neutrophil peptides 1–3. Int J Tuberc Lung Dis 15:369–374
211. Okada M, Kita Y, Nakajima T, Kanamaru N, Hashimoto S, Nagasawa T, Kaneda Y, Yoshida S, Nishida Y, Nakatani H, Takao K, Kishigami C, Nishimatsu S, Sekine Y, Inoue Y, Matsumoto M, McMurray DN, De la Cruz EC, Tan EV, Abalos RM, Burgos JA, Saunderson P, Sakatani M (2011) Novel therapeutic vaccine: granulysin and new DNA vaccine against tuberculosis. Hum Vaccin Immunother 7:S60–S67
212. Nemeth E, Ganz T (2009) The role of hepcidin in iron metabolism. Acta Haematol 122:78–86
213. Yang H, Chen H, Liu Z, Ma H, Qin L, Jin RL, Zheng R, Feng Y, Cui Z, Wang J, Liu J, Hu Z (2013) A novel B-cell epitope identified within Mycobacterium tuberculosis CFP10/ESAT-6 protein. PLoS One 8:e52848
214. Alonso S, Pethe K, Russell DG, Purdy GE (2007) Lysosomal killing of Mycobacterium mediated by ubiquitin-derived peptides is enhanced by autophagy. Proc Natl Acad Sci U S A 104:6031–6036
215. Foss MH, Powers KM, Purdy GE (2012) Structural and functional characterization of mycobactericidal ubiquitin-derived peptides in model and bacterial membranes. Biochemistry 51:9922–9929
216. Chung HJ, Montville TJ, Chikindas ML (2000) Nisin depletes ATP and proton motive force in mycobacteria. Lett Appl Microbiol 31:416–420
217. Carroll J, Draper LA, O'Connor PM, Coffey A, Hill C, Ross RP, Cotter PD, O'Mahony J (2010) Comparison of the activities of the lantibiotics nisin and lacticin 3147 against clinically significant mycobacteria. Int J Antimicrob Agents 36:132–136
218. Bagley MC, Dale JW, Merritt EA, Xiong X (2005) Thiopeptide antibiotics. Chem Rev 105:685–714
219. Koyama N, Kojima S, Nonaka K, Masuma R, Matsumoto M, Omura S, Tomoda H (2010) Calpinactam, a new anti-mycobacterial agent, produced by Mortierella alpina FKI-4905. J Antibiot 63:183–186
220. Pruksakorn P, Arai M, Kotoku N, Vilcheze C, Baughn AD, Moodley P, Jacobs WR Jr, Kobayashi M (2010) Tri-choderins, novel aminolipopeptides from a marine sponge-derived Trichoderma sp., are active against dormant mycobacteria. Bioorg Med Chem Lett 20:3658–3663

221. Haritakun R, Sappan M, Suvannakad R, Tasanathai K, Isaka M (2010) An antimycobacterial cyclodepsipeptide from the entomopathogenic fungus Ophiocordyceps communis BCC 16475. J Nat Prod 73:75–78
222. Aarti C, Khusro A (2013) Snake venom as Anticancer agent- current perspective. Int J Pure Appl Biosci 1:24–29
223. Xie JP, Yue J, Xiong YL, Wang WY, Yu SQ, Wang HH (2003) In vitro activities of small peptides from snake venom against clinical isolates of drug-resistant Mycobacterium tuberculosis. Int J Antimicrob Agents 22:172–174
224. Bhunia SK, Sarkar M, Dey S, Bhakta A, Gomes A, Giri B (2015) *In vitro* activity screening of snake venom against multi drug resistant tuberculosis. Int J Trop Dis 4:1–4
225. Rodriguez A, Villegas E, Montoya-Rosales A, Rivas-Santiago B, Corzo G (2014) Characterization of antibacterial and hemolytic activity of synthetic Pandinin 2 variants and their inhibition against Mycobacterium tuberculosis. PLoS One 9:e101742

Lung Cancer: Pathophysiology and Current Advancements in Therapeutics

6

Prabhu Thirusangu and V. Vigneshwaran

Abstract

Lung cancer, a highly invasive, rapidly metastasizing and prevalent cancer, is the top killer malignancy in both men and women in the United States of America (USA), Europe, United Kingdom (UK), and developing Asian countries. Lung cancer causes more deaths per year than the next four leading cancers (colon/rectal, breast, pancreas, and prostate) together in the United States. However, over the last two decades, we have observed enhanced outcomes that are mostly attributable to initial detection, improved efforts in tobacco control, amended surgical approaches, and the development of novel targeted therapies. At present, there are numerous novel therapies in clinical practice, including those targeting actionable mutations and more lately immunotherapeutic drugs. Immunotherapy signifies the most noteworthy step forward in eliminating this deadly disease. This chapter highlights the major advances in treatments with therapeutic intent, systemic targeted therapies, comforting care, and early detection in lung cancer. We discuss the fundamental research that reinforces these new technologies/strategies and their current position in clinical practice.

Keywords

Lung cancer · Immunotherapy · Chemotherapy · Radiation · Targeted therapy

Prabhu and Vigneshwaran contributed equally to this work.

P. Thirusangu (✉)
Department of Experimental Pathology and Medicine, Mayo Clinic, Rochester, MN, USA
e-mail: thirusangu.prabhu@mayo.edu

V. Vigneshwaran
Department of Pharmacology, Centre for Lung and Vascular Biology, University of Illinois at Chicago, Chicago, IL, USA

S. Rayees et al. (eds.), *Chronic Lung Diseases*,
https://doi.org/10.1007/978-981-15-3734-9_6

Abbreviations

DNMTs	DNA methyltransferases
HDAC	Histone deacetylases
NSCLC	Non-small-cell lung cancer
PD-1	Programmed cell death receptor 1
PD-L1	Programmed cell death receptor ligand 1
SCLC	Small-cell lung cancer

6.1 Introduction

The fundamental abnormality resulting in the development of cancer is the continual unregulated proliferation of cancer cells. Rather than responding appropriately to the signals that control normal cell behavior, cancer cells grow and divide in an uncontrolled manner, invading normal tissues and organs and eventually spreading throughout the body. At the cellular level, the development of cancer is viewed as a multistep process involving mutation and selection for cells with progressively increasing capacity for proliferation, survival, invasion, and metastasis [1]. William Osler, in his 1912 edition of his classic textbook of medicine, stated that "primary tumors of the lung are rare" [2]. But today, lung cancer is the commonly diagnosed malignancy and the leading cause of cancer death in the world. It has been transformed from a rare disease into a global problem and public health issue. The etiologic factors of lung cancer become more complex along with industrialization, urbanization, and environmental pollution around the world [3, 4].

Sir Austin Bradford Hill is a pioneering epidemiologist who established the link between smoking and lung cancer. By the mid-1940s, the rate of lung cancer was increasing at epidemic proportions, but the cause was unknown. Austin Bradford Hill and Richard Doll designed a comprehensive epidemiological study to investigate the effects of a wide variety of exposures that were new at that time, which included automobile exhaust, road tars, atmospheric pollution, and cigarette smoking. Doll and Hill found cigarette smoking as a single most cause that was correlated with the higher incidence of lung cancer. This landmark study concluded that smoking as a potent carcinogen in 1950s [5–7]. Even today, lung cancer continues to be an unabating pandemic. One in ten tobacco smokers develops bronchogenic carcinoma over a lifetime. Unless further reductions in the prevalence of cigarette smoking are achieved over the next decade, lung cancer is predicted to remain as an all too common, but avoidable, disease [8, 9].

Lung cancer, although highly preventable, is usually diagnosed at an incurable stage. Chemotherapy is playing an increasingly important role alongside surgery and radiation therapy in the management of this disease [10]. Despite the efficacy of chemotherapeutic drugs, an important factor for the failure of many agents is the primary or acquired resistance to therapy. This is inexplicably explained by intratumoral heterogeneity that includes genetic mutations, interactions with the microenvironment, and the presence of cancer stem cells [11]. Therefore, future advances in understanding and treating lung cancer will be based on genetic analysis.

This review will focus on the epidemiology, etiologic factors contributing to the development of the lung cancer, biology of the disease, and the current treatment modalities. As last decade has witnessed rapid advances in the immune checkpoint inhibitors, this review will also summarize the modern advancements in the immunotherapy and targeted therapies.

6.1.1 Epidemiology/Morbidity

Lung cancer has been the most common cancer worldwide since 1985, in terms of both incidence and mortality. Globally, lung cancer is the largest contributor to new cancer diagnoses (1,350,000 new cases and 12.4% of total new cancer cases) and cancer deaths (1,180,000 deaths and 17.6% of total cancer deaths) [12, 13]. Lung cancer rates vary around the world, reflecting geographical differences in tobacco use and air quality. They also vary substantially by sex, age, race/ethnicity, and socioeconomic status [4].

There has been a large relative increase in the numbers of lung cancer cases in developing countries. Approximately half (49.9%) of the cases now occur in developing countries, whereas in 1980, 69% of cases were in developed countries. The estimated numbers of lung cancer cases worldwide have increased by 51% since 1985 (a 44% increase in men and a 76% increase in women) [12, 13]. Epidemiological studies of lung cancer among nonsmoking men are few. A study indicated that occupational carcinogens and indoor radon may play a role in some lung cancers in nonsmoking men [14].

6.1.2 Etiology of Lung Cancer

Harting and Hesse in 1879 reported the first description of occupational lung cancer. They reported the association between lung cancer and work in the Schneeberg mines in Germany. Subsequent studies early in twentieth century indicated high levels of radon gas found in the mines and an etiologic connection between radioactive gas exposure and development of lung carcinogeneis [15].

In research carried out over the last half of the twentieth century, many factors were causally associated with lung cancer, and studies were implemented to identify determinants of susceptibility to these factors. The major risk factor for lung cancer is smoking that accounts for 75–80% of lung cancer-related deaths. It is identified as the single most predominant cause of the lung cancer epidemic. But other important causes include workplace agents (e.g., asbestos, arsenic, chromium, nickel, and radon) and other environmental factors (passive smoking, indoor radon, and air pollution) [8]. Smoking increases lung cancer risk five- to tenfold with a clear dose–

Table 6.1 Classification of lung tumors

S. No.	Type	Percentage of all lung cancers	Anatomic location
Non-small-cell lung carcinoma			
1	Squamous cell lung cancers (SQCLC)	25–30%	Arise in main bronchi and advance to the carina
2	Adenocarcinomas (AdenoCA)	40%	Arise in peripheral bronchi
3	Large-cell anaplastic carcinomas (LCAC)	10%	Tumors lack the classic glandular or squamous morphology
Small-cell lung carcinoma			
1	Small-cell lung carcinoma cancers (SCLC)	10–15%	Derive from the hormonal cells; disseminate into submucosal lymphatic vessels and regional lymph nodes almost without a bronchial invasion

response relationship. Exposure to environmental tobacco smoke among nonsmokers increases lung cancer risk about 20% [16].

Apart from the smoking and chemical agents, viral infections also play vital part in the development of lung cancer. Large-cell lymphoepithelial lung carcinoma, a rare variant of large-cell carcinoma, is associated with the Epstein–Barr virus. Human papillomaviruses (HPV) have also been associated with the development of lung cancer. There are notable geographical differences, however. In Germany, maximum HPV detection rates of 4.2% have been reported, whereas in certain regions of Asia, these were as high as 80% [17, 18].

6.2 Pathophysiology of Lung Cancer

6.2.1 Biology of the Disease

Lung cancer arises from the cells of the respiratory epithelium. It is divided into two broad histologic classes, which grow and spread differently: small-cell lung carcinomas (SCLCs) and non-small-cell lung carcinomas (NSCLCs) (Table 6.1) [13, 19, 20]. Small-cell lung cancer (SCLC) is a highly malignant tumor derived from cells exhibiting neuroendocrine characteristics and accounts for 15% of lung cancer cases. Non-small-cell lung cancer (NSCLC), which accounts for the remaining 85% of cases, is further divided into three major pathologic subtypes: adenocarcinoma, squamous cell carcinoma, and large-cell carcinoma. Adenocarcinoma alone accounts for 38.5% of all lung cancer cases, with squamous cell carcinoma accounting for 20% and large-cell carcinoma accounting for 2.9% [13, 19, 21].

6.2.1.1 Small-Cell Lung Cancer

Small-cell lung cancer (SCLC) is an aggressive cancer of neuroendocrine origin, which is strongly associated with cigarette smoking. Patients typically present with a short duration of symptoms and frequently (60–65%) with metastatic disease [22]. Compared with non-small-cell lung cancers (NSCLC), SCLC is characterized by a rapid doubling time and early, widespread metastases. Consequently, most patients (60–70%) will have extensive-stage (ES) disease at the time of diagnosis (defined as cancer that has spread beyond the ipsilateral lung and regional lymph nodes and cannot be included in a single radiation field) [23].

6.2.1.2 Non-Small-Cell Lung Cancer

Clinically, non-small-cell lung cancer (NSCLC) accounts for around 85% of total lung cancers, with adenocarcinoma (AC; 40%) and squamous cell carcinoma (SCC; 30%) representing the major sub-histotypes. Lesions containing both AC and SCC features are classified as adenosquamous carcinoma (ASC; 0.4–4%), a rare disease with poor prognosis [24–26].

6.2.2 Molecular Epidemiology of Lung Cancer

Technologic advances over the last 20 years have allowed for the investigation of the molecular mechanisms underlying susceptibility to lung cancer and provided the necessary tools for molecular epidemiology studies. Susceptibility differences may be inherited in the form of low-frequency, high-penetrance genes or high-frequency, low-penetrance genes or may be acquired through epigenetic mechanisms such as methylation, with likely genetic heterogeneity [27]. New insights into lung carcinogenesis have made the study of molecular markers of risk possible in human populations in the emerging field of molecular epidemiology. Recent data have addressed the relationships of human lung cancer to polymorphisms of phase I procarcinogen-activating and phase II deactivating enzymes and intermediate biomarkers of DNA mutation, such as DNA adducts, oncogene and tumor suppressor gene mutations, and polymorphisms [9].

Malignant cells are well documented to reprogram their metabolism and energy production networks to support rapid proliferation and survival in harsh conditions via mutations in oncogenes and inactivation of tumor suppressor genes [27, 28]. Lung cancer cells often harbor mutations in genes and pathways, such as the PI3K (phosphoinositide-3-kinase)-AKT-mTOR (mammalian target of rapamycin) pathway, the oncogenes RAS, c-MYC, and HIF-1 (hypoxia inducible factor), and the tumor suppressor gene TP53 (tumor protein) [28].

The epigenome consists of heritable modifications of DNA, histones, and chromatin that may act to modulate gene expression independently of DNA coding alterations. Epigenetic changes such as global DNA hypomethylation, regional DNA hypermethylation, and aberrant histone modification, each influence the expression of oncogenes and lead to the development and progression of tumors. Crucially, epigenetic dysregulation, unlike genetic mutations, may be reversed by selectively targeted therapies. Epigenetic modifications that may be readily targeted with currently available therapies include regional DNA hypermethylation and histone hypoacetylation with hypomethylating agents and histone deacetylase inhibitors (HDI), respectively.

6.3 Current Treatment Modalities

Treatment options for lung cancer include surgery, radiation therapy, chemotherapy, and targeted therapy. Therapeutic modalities recommendations depend on several factors, including the type and stage of cancer. The diagnosis of the malignancy is done by chest radiography, sputum cytology, bronchoscopy, needle biopsy, and other techniques. Drugs targeting ALK, ROS, and the EGF and VEGF pathways have been particularly beneficial for patients with nonsquamous NSCLCs. However, we have learnt that—after dramatic initial responses—the long-term effects of the target cancer therapies are limited mainly by acquired resistance. So, searching for new therapeutic options always warrants efforts [10, 29].

6.3.1 Surgery and Radiation

Surgical resection remains the single most consistent and successful treatment of choice for early stage, localized lung tumors. For this option to be feasible, the cancer must be completely resectable, and the patient must be able to tolerate the proposed surgical intervention (Table 6.2) [30–32]. Lobectomy has been the gold standard for the resection of early-stage NSCLC since the Lung Cancer Study Group trial results were published in 1995. But approximately 25% of patients with early-stage NSCLC are not candidates for lobectomy, the preferred surgical procedure, because of severe medical comorbidities [33].

Although there were no differences in perioperative morbidity or mortality between the groups, patients with limited resection (either wedge resection or segmentectomy) experienced a significantly higher incidence of disease recurrence, perhaps because of occult nodal metastases, which may be present in 4–20% of patients undergoing resection of clinical stage I lung cancer [33, 34]. Wedge resection is a nonanatomic resection in which interlobar and parenchymal (N1) lymph

Table 6.2 Types of lung surgery to treat NSCLC

S. No.	Type of surgery	Description
1	Pneumonectomy	Removal of the entire lung
2	Segmentectomy or wedge resection	Surgery involving the removal of the section of lobe.
3	Lobectomy	Surgical removal of the entire lobe
4	Sleeve resection or sleeve lobectomy	Lobe of the lung and a part of the bronchi are removed

nodes are not typically obtained for pathologic analysis. In contrast, both segmentectomy and lobectomy are anatomic lung resections in which these nodes are identified and removed for a more accurate pathologic staging. The 3- and 5-year overall survival rates after open lobectomy have been shown to be approximately 82% and 66%, respectively [30, 31].

Nowadays, minimal-access surgical procedures are expanding the applicability of surgical resection to patients of marginal operability. Video-assisted thoracic surgery lobectomy provides a less invasive method of accomplishing the oncologic resection with long-term survival rate [32, 35]. After surgery, adjuvant chemotherapy is prescribed to lower the risk of recurrence in patients with lymph node involvement [29, 36].

6.3.1.1 Radiation Therapy

Radiotherapy is the most important nonsurgical modality for the curative treatment of cancer. High-energy radiation damages genetic material (deoxyribonucleic acid, DNA) of cells and thus blocking their ability to divide and proliferate further. Although radiation damages both normal cells as well as cancer cells, the goal of radiation therapy is to maximize the radiation dose to abnormal cancer cells while minimizing exposure to normal cells, which is adjacent to cancer cells or in the path of radiation. Radiation therapy remains an important component of cancer treatment with approximately 50% of all cancer patients receiving radiation therapy during their course of illness; it contributes towards 40% of curative treatment for cancer [37, 38].

6.3.1.2 Stereotactic Body Radiation Therapy (SBRT)

SBRT is a complex radiation technique that requires not only sophisticated treatment planning and delivery systems but also a radiation oncologist proficient in SBRT procedures. The fundamental difference between SBRT and conventional radiation therapy is the utilization of substantially larger doses during each treatment session. For comparison, a conventional daily dose of radiation therapy is 2 Gy, which is typically given 5 days a week for approximately 6 weeks. A typical SBRT course for stage I NSCLC consists of 1–5 treatments over a 1- to 2-week time period with daily doses of 10–34 Gy. Not only is SBRT more convenient for patients because of the shorter treatment duration, but also the larger doses make SBRT more biologically potent and lead to high rates of local tumor control. Indeed, prospective studies have consistently shown 3-year local control rates of approximately 90% with SBRT for stage I NSCLC [30]. Most patients tolerate SBRT exceptionally well. Mild fatigue, lasting for 1–2 weeks after treatment completion, is common [30, 39].

6.3.2 Chemotherapy and Immunotherapy

Despite great effort in encouraging screening or, at least, a close surveillance of high-risk individuals, most of lung cancers are diagnosed when already surgically

Table 6.3 List of latest FDA-approved therapeutic drugs for NSCLCs [29]

S. No.	FDA-approved drugs	Target protein	Category
1	Crizotinib	ALK-1 ROS1	First-line therapy
2	Afatinib	EGFR HER2	First-line therapy
3	Bevacizumab	VEGF	First-line therapy
4	Ceritinib Alectinib Brigatinib	ALK-1	Second-line therapy
5	Osimertinib	EGFR (T790M)	Second-line therapy
6	Ramucirumab	VEGFR2	Second-line therapy

unresectable because of local advancement or metastasis. In these cases, the treatment of choice is chemotherapy, alone or in combination with radiotherapy [29].

Chemotherapy is also the only palliative, systemic treatment for metastatic tumors. Finally, chemotherapy is the treatment of choice for patients who, regardless of tumor stage, are not eligible for lung resection because of their respiratory and/or general status. Thus, overall, more than 80% of newly diagnosed lung cancer patients receive chemotherapy, alone or in combination with radiotherapy. The combination of carboplatin and paclitaxel has long been the most common first-line therapeutic regimen prescribed for NSCLCs. Docetaxel, gemcitabine, vinorelbine, irinotecan, and topotecan combinations have also shown some promise [10]. However, in the last few years, NSCLC treatment has been dramatically changed by the FDA approval of many new target therapies (Table 6.3).

6.3.2.1 Immunotherapy

Several seminal events in modern immunology set the stage for the translation of immunologic concepts into effective immunotherapies for cancer [40]. Dysfunctional tumor immune interactions leading to immune evasion are key events in tumorigenesis and metastasis [41]. Vital factors related to immune escape include the lack of strong cancer antigens or epitopes recognized by T cells, minimal activation of cancer-specific T cells, poor infiltration of T cells into tumors, downregulation of the major histocompatibility complex on cancer cells, and immunosuppressive factors and cells in the tumor microenvironment [42]. The clinical goal of tumor immunotherapy is to provide either passive or active immunity against malignancies by harnessing the immune system to target tumors [43]. The very recent approval of drugs targeting the PD-L1/PD-1 pathway has been a groundbreaking advancement especially for the treatment of squamous NSCLCs. Physiologically, PD-1 is expressed on regulatory and cytotoxic-activated T cells. Binding of PD-L1 to its receptor inactivates the T cells, a key mechanism to limit immune responses [44]. PD-1 is highly expressed on many tumor-infiltrating lymphocytes, but cancer cells often overexpress PD-L1, so blocking the immune attack against themselves. This has provided a strong rationale for the development of drugs targeting the PD-1 pathway. Indeed, drugs blocking the binding of PD-L1 to its receptor, such as nivolumab and pembrolizumab, enhance immunity against a wide variety of cancers, including NSCLC [29].

6.3.3 Epigenetic Therapy

The involvement of epigenetic alterations in the evolution of different cancers has led to the development of epigenetics-based therapies, mainly targeting DNA methyltransferases (DNMTs) and histone-modifying enzymes [45].

6.3.3.1 DNA Methyltransferase Inhibitors: Single-Agent Studies

Decitabine and 5-azacytidine are cytosine analogues that act to inhibit DNMT and consequently DNA methylation. Decitabine is a deoxyribonucleotide that is directly incorporated into DNA, thus inhibiting DNA methylation, whereas azacytidine is a ribonucleotide precursor that has approximately 10% of the potency of decitabine. Although their regulatory approvals to date have been in hematologic malignancies, several clinical trials of single-agent therapy have been conducted in solid tumors that included NSCLC [46].

Between 1972 and 1977, 103 patients with NSCLC received single-agent azacytidine on seven different solid tumor clinical protocols; however, efficacy proved extremely limited with an objective response rate of only 8%. Similarly, more than 200 patients with NSCLC have been enrolled on clinical trials of single-agent decitabine with only two objective responses reported. These disappointing initial findings have led further to the investigation of combinatorial therapies, in particular concurrent epigenetic therapy with HDIs [46].

6.3.3.2 Histone-Modifying Enzymes

Two HDIs have been FDA approved to date, vorinostat (SAHA) and romidepsin (depsipeptide), for use in cutaneous and peripheral T-cell lymphomas. It is unknown at present whether the strategy of using highly selective agents is better than broader targeting of multiple HDAC isoforms in lung cancer. HDIs have been demonstrated to have a multitude of anticancer effects, including causing G_1 cell-cycle arrest via activation of p21 and decreasing cyclin expression, ultimately leading to the activation of apoptotic pathways. Additional effects include downregulation of checkpoint kinase 1, suppression of proangiogenic and matrix remodeling genes, and activation of T cells and natural killer cells by upregulating MHC classes I and II, CD80/CD86, and MICA/MICB. Clinically, the use of single-agent HDIs in patients with previously treated advanced NSCLC has yielded disappointing results with disease stabilization rather than objective response being the main effect. Although HDI monotherapy does not seem to be a successful strategy in NSCLC, there is promise that when combined with demethylating agents, the multitargeting approach may have more activity [45, 46].

Table 6.4 Adverse effects of radiation therapy

Type	Duration	Pathogenesis
Acute toxicity This is usually observed in rapidly proliferating tissues such as skin, gastrointestinal tract and the hematopoietic system.	Occurs during or within weeks of treatment. Usually reversible and not generally considered dose-limiting.	Example: bone marrow suppression, dermatitis, mucositis, cystitis, proctitis, and hair loss.
Late toxicity Late effects typically occur in more slowly proliferating tissues, such as kidney, heart and central nervous system.	Occurring 6 months to many years later. As late side effects can be permanent, they provide the basis for dose constraints to radiation toxicity.	Fibrosis, hormone deficiency, infertility, vascular damage, and second malignancy.

6.4 Drawbacks of the Current Treatment

Survival rate after a lung cancer diagnosis has changed little, with overall 5-year relative survival rate increasing only slightly from 12.4% for 1974–1976 diagnoses to 15.0% for 1996–2002 diagnoses. This slight improvement in survival rate reflects limited advances in screening and treatment for lung cancer (Table 6.4) [47].

6.4.1 Surgical Morbidity

Although surgery remains the successful treatment of choice for the treatment of lung cancer, surgical morbidity is one of the undesirable outcome in the current treatment. The incidence of major morbidity after surgery, which includes a composite of cardiopulmonary outcomes such as pneumonia, respiratory failure, myocardial infarction, and unexpected returns to the operating room, is approximately 9%.

6.4.2 Radiation Toxicity

Although the functional and structural tolerance of normal tissue to radiotherapy is contextual, studies of cell and tissue response to ionizing radiation have led to an improved understanding of the pathogenesis of radiation toxicity. Recent radiobiology research suggests that normal tissue injury is a dynamic and progressive process. The deposition of energy results in DNA damage and changes in the microenvironment through chemokines, inflammatory cytokines, fibrotic cytokines, altered cell–cell interactions, influx of inflammatory cells, and the induction of reparative and restorative processes (Table 6.4) [37, 48].

Despite recent great advances in the identification of novel targetable genetic lesions and in the development of new drugs, lung cancer is still the leading cause of cancer-related mortality: thus, one of the major human killers with a disappointing 5-year survival rate of 15% [29, 49]. It is, therefore, literally vital to search for new drugs or to improve the current treatment protocols to increase efficacy, overcome resistance, and reduce side effects.

6.5 Future Directions in Therapeutics

Epigenetic modifications play an important role in the development and progression of NSCLC. Recent data on the use of gene methylation as a prognostic marker for early-stage NSCLC are promising and may help to direct efforts toward targeted epigenetic therapy as adjuvant therapy. On the basis of the results obtained in NSCLC- and SCLC-derived cell lines and in tumor samples, a recent report indicated CCDC6 as a biomarker for a more personalized lung cancer therapy [29].

Standard chemotherapeutic regimens have devastating effects on the patient's immune system. Recent developments in immunology indicate that immunostimulatory perspectives have significant implications in the design of dynamic immunotherapeutic strategies for treating malignancies such as lung cancer. Several plant-derived compounds such as flavonoids, polysaccharides, lactones, alkaloids, diterpenoids, glycosides, and lectins have been reported to be responsible for the immunomodulatory properties [50, 51]. Thus, future investigations expediting molecular insights of immunopotentiating plant-derived compounds would provide novel leads in the development of potent and safe cancer therapeutics. Apart from the efficacy, specific immunomodulatory agents from plant origin also possess potential to counteract the side effects and high cost of synthetic compounds. Anti-tumor vaccines and dendritic cell-based therapies are recently emerging as novel and potent inducers of immune response against the tumor.

References

1. Cooper GM (2000) The cell: a molecular approach. The development and causes of cancer, 2nd edn. Sinauer Associates, Sunderland, MA
2. Miller YE (2005) Pathogenesis of lung cancer: 100 year report. Am J Respir Cell Mol Biol 33:216–223
3. Mao Y, Yang D, He J, Krasna MJ (2016) Epidemiology of lung cancer. Surg Oncol Clin N Am 25:439–445
4. Torre LA, Siegel RL, Jemal A (2016) Lung cancer statistics. Adv Exp Med Biol 893:1–19
5. Doll R, Hill AB (1950) Smoking and carcinoma of the lung; preliminary report. Br Med J 2:739–748
6. Doll R (1991) Conversation with Sir Richard Doll. Br J Addict 86:365–377
7. Blackadar CB (2016) Historical review of the causes of cancer. World J Clin Oncol 7:54–86
8. Alberg AJ, Brock MV, Samet JM (2005) Epidemiology of lung cancer: looking to the future. J Clin Oncol 23:3175–3185

9. Spivack SD, Fasco MJ, Walker VE, Kaminsky LS (1997) The molecular epidemiology of lung cancer. Crit Rev Toxicol 27:319–365
10. Cersosimo RJ (2002) Lung cancer: a review. Am J Health Syst Pharm 59:611–642
11. Dawood S, Austin L, Cristofanilli M (2014) Cancer stem cells: implications for cancer therapy. Oncology (Williston Park) 28:1101–1110
12. Siegel R, Ward E, Brawley O, Jemal A (2011) Cancer statistics, 2011: the impact of eliminating socioeconomic and racial disparities on premature cancer deaths. CA Cancer J Clin 61:212–236
13. Dela Cruz CS, Tanoue LT, Matthay RA (2011) Lung cancer: epidemiology, etiology, and prevention. Clin Chest Med 32:605–644
14. Kreuzer M, Gerken M, Kreienbrock L, Wellmann J, Wichmann HE (2001) Lung cancer in lifetime nonsmoking men - results of a case-control study in Germany. Br J Cancer 84:134–140
15. Greenberg M, Selikoff IJ (1993) Lung cancer in the Schneeberg mines: a reappraisal of the data reported by Harting and Hesse in 1879. Ann Occup Hyg 37:5–14
16. Schwartz AG, Cote ML (2016) Epidemiology of lung cancer. Adv Exp Med Biol 893:21–41
17. Petersen I (2011) The morphological and molecular diagnosis of lung cancer. Dtsch Arztebl Int 108(31-32):525–531
18. Klein F, Amin Kotb WF, Petersen I (2009) Incidence of human papilloma virus in lung cancer. Lung Cancer 65:13–18
19. Howlader N, Noone AM, Krapcho M et al (eds) (2010) SEER cancer statistics review, 1975–2008. National Cancer Institute, Bethesda, MD
20. Lemjabbar-Alaoui H, Hassan OU, Yang YW, Buchanan P (2015) Lung cancer: biology and treatment options. Biochim Biophys Acta 1856:189–210
21. Herbst RS, Heymach JV, Lippman SM (2008) Lung cancer. N Engl J Med 359:1367–1380
22. Bernhardt EB, Jalal SI (2016) Small cell lung cancer. Cancer Treat Res 170:301–322
23. Byers LA, Rudin CM (2015) Small cell lung cancer: where do we go from here? Cancer 121:664–672
24. Nagaraj AS, Lahtela J, Hemmes A et al (2017) Cell of origin links histotype spectrum to immune microenvironment diversity in non-small-cell lung cancer driven by mutant kras and loss of Lkb1. Cell Rep 18:673–684
25. Nakagawa K, Yasumitu T, Fukuhara K, Shiono H, Kikui M (2003) Poor prognosis after lung resection for patients with adenosquamous carcinoma of the lung. Ann Thorac Surg 75:1740–1744
26. Travis WD, Brambilla E, Riely GJ (2013) New pathologic classification of lung cancer: relevance for clinical practice and clinical trials. J Clin Oncol 31:992–1001
27. Ann GS, Geoffrey MP, Cathryn HB, Michele LC (2007) The molecular epidemiology of lung cancer. Carcinogenesis 28:507–518
28. Karolien V, Geert-Jan G, Liesbet M, Michiel T, Elien D, Jean-Paul N, Wanda G, Peter A (2019) The metabolic landscape of lung cancer: new insights in a disturbed glucose metabolism. Front Oncol 9:1215
29. Visconti R, Morra F, Guggino G, Celetti A (2017) The between now and then of lung cancer chemotherapy and immunotherapy. Int J Mol Sci 18:1374
30. Tandberg DJ, Tong BC, Ackerson BG, Kelsey CR (2018) Surgery versus stereotactic body radiation therapy for stage I non-small cell lung cancer: a comprehensive review. Cancer 124:667–678
31. Donington J, Ferguson M, Mazzone P et al (2012) American College of Chest Physicians and Society of Thoracic Surgeons consensus statement for evaluation and management for high risk patients with stage I non–small cell lung cancer. Chest 142:1620–1635
32. Molina JR, Yang P, Cassivi SD, Schild SE, Adjei AA (2008) Non-small cell lung cancer: epidemiology, risk factors, treatment, and survivorship. Mayo Clin Proc 83:584–594
33. Kohman LJ, Gu L, Altorki N et al (2017) Biopsy first: lessons learned from Cancer and Leukemia Group B (CALGB). J Thorac Cardiovasc Surg 153:1592–1597

34. Martin P, Shiau CJ, Pasic M, Tsao M, Kamel-Reid S, Lin S et al (2016) Clinical impact of mutation fraction in epidermal growth factor receptor mutation positive NSCLC patients. Br J Cancer 114:616–622
35. McKenna RJ Jr, Houck W, Fuller CB (2006) Video-assisted thoracic surgery lobectomy: experience with 1,100 cases. Ann Thorac Surg 81:421–426
36. Lackey A, Donington JS (2013) Surgical management of lung cancer. Semin Interv Radiol 30:133–140
37. Barnett GC, West CM, Dunning AM et al (2009) Normal tissue reactions to radiotherapy: towards tailoring treatment dose by genotype. Nat Rev Cancer 9:134–142
38. Baskar R, Lee KA, Yeo R, Yeoh KW (2012) Cancer and radiation therapy: current advances and future directions. Int J Med Sci 9:193–199
39. Timmerman R, Paulus R, Galvin J et al (2010) Stereotactic body radiation therapy for inoperable early stage lung cancer. JAMA 303:1070–1076
40. Rosenberg SA (2014) IL-2: the first effective immunotherapy for human cancer. J Immunol 192:5451–5458
41. Hanahan D, Weinberg RA (2011) Hallmarks of cancer: the next generation. Cell 144:646–674
42. Kim JM, Chen DS (2016) Immune escape to PD-L1/PD-1 blockade: seven steps to success (or failure). Ann Oncol 27:1492–1504
43. Baxevanis CN, Perez SA, Papamichail M (2009) Cancer immunotherapy. Crit Rev Clin Lab Sci 46:167–189
44. Yao S, Chen L (2014) PD-1 as an immune modulatory receptor. Cancer J 20:262–264
45. Schiffmann I, Greve G, Jung M, Lübbert M (2016) Epigenetic therapy approaches in non-small cell lung cancer: update and perspectives. Epigenetics 11:858–870
46. Forde PM, Brahmer JR, Kelly RJ (2014) New strategies in lung cancer: epigenetic therapy for non-small cell lung cancer. Clin Cancer Res 20:2244–2248
47. Ries LAG et al (2004) SEER cancer statistics review, 1975-2001. National Cancer Institute, Bethesda, MD
48. Bentzen SM (2006) Preventing or reducing late side effects of radiation therapy: radiobiology meets molecular pathology. Nat Rev Cancer 6:702–713
49. Siegel RL, Miller KD, Jemal A (2017) Cancer statistics. CA Cancer J Clin 67:7–30
50. Vigneshwaran V, Thirusangu P, Vijay Avin BR, Krishna V, Pramod SN, Prabhakar BT (2017) Immunomodulatory glc/man-directed Dolichos lablab lectin (DLL) evokes anti-tumour response in vivo by counteracting angiogenic gene expressions. Clin Exp Immunol 189:21–35
51. Jantan I, Ahmad W, Bukhari SN (2015) Plant-derived immunomodulators: an insight on their preclinical evaluation and clinical trials. Front Plant Sci 6:655

Acute Respiratory Distress Syndrome: Therapeutics, Pathobiology, and Prognosis

7

Vigneshwaran Vellingiri, Prabhu Thirusangu, and Inshah Din

Abstract

Acute respiratory distress syndrome (ARDS) is a critical syndrome consisting of acute respiratory failure, which is characterized by injury to the alveolar capillary barrier that leads to the influx of protein-rich fluid infiltrates into alveolar spaces and subsequent devastating lung fibrosis. This deadly respiratory condition can be caused by various pulmonary (e.g., pneumonia, aspiration) or non-pulmonary (e.g., sepsis, pancreatitis, trauma) injuries, leading to the development of nonhydrostatic pulmonary edema. Despite various seminal events in the understanding of molecular mechanisms underpinning the ARDS, the armamentarium of therapies aimed at the underlying pathology remains limited and highly ineffective. ARDS has an enormous mortality rate of approximately 40%. Till today, ARDS management remains mostly supportive with lung-protective mechanical ventilation. Here, we deduce the recent advances in the understanding of the biology of the disease, the diagnosis, and the treatment of ARDS. Moreover, this review also provides a historical background and highlights areas of future perspectives in therapeutics.

Keywords

ARDS · Alveolar capillary barrier · Fibrosis · Pneumonia · Sepsis · Pancreatitis · Trauma · Mechanical ventilation

V. Vellingiri (✉)
Department of Pharmacology, Center for Lung and Vascular Biology, University of Illinois at Chicago, Chicago, IL, USA
e-mail: vigneshw@uic.edu

P. Thirusangu
Department of Experimental Pathology and Medicine, Mayo Clinic, Rochester, MN, USA

I. Din
Department of Biochemistry, Govt. Medical College Srinagar, Srinagar, India

S. Rayees et al. (eds.), *Chronic Lung Diseases*,
https://doi.org/10.1007/978-981-15-3734-9_7

7.1 Introduction

The syndrome of acute respiratory distress (ARDS) is a life-threatening condition that is characterized by intense lung inflammation, diffuse alveolar damage, progressive micro-atelectasis, increased pulmonary vascular permeability, increased lung weight, and loss of aerated tissue [1, 2]. ARDS was first described in 1967 by Ashbaugh et al. [3] in a case series of 12 patients who shared the common features of unusually persistent tachypnea and hypoxemia, opacification on chest radiographs, and poor lung compliance, despite different underlying causes [2–4].

Following the initial description of acute respiratory distress syndrome (ARDS) by Ashbaugh et al. in 1967, multiple definitions were proposed and used until the 1994 publication of the American-European Consensus Conference (AECC) definition. The AECC defined ARDS as the acute onset of hypoxemia (arterial partial pressure of oxygen to a fraction of inspired oxygen [PaO2/FIO2] 200 mmHg) with bilateral infiltrates on frontal chest radiographs, with no evidence of left atrial hypertension. A new overarching entity—acute lung injury (ALI)—was also described, using similar criteria but with less severe hypoxemia (PaO2/FIO2 300 mmHg) [5].

Initially, ARDS was described as an "adult" respiratory distress syndrome to differentiate it from infant respiratory distress syndrome. Presently, this has been changed to acute respiratory distress syndrome due to the fact that both adults and children develop ARDS. Lung development increases linearly with age and height until the adolescent growth spurt at 10 years in girls and 12 years in boys. Therefore, there are significant differences between adult and child ARDS pathophysiology due to remodeling, growth of the lung parenchyma, and progressive maturation of the immune system [5–10]. Until recently, the most widely accepted definition was that from the American European Consensus Conference (AECC) in 1994. The AECC defined ARDS as the acute onset of hypoxemia with bilateral infiltrates on a frontal chest radiograph, with no clinical evidence of left atrial hypertension (or pulmonary artery wedge pressure of greater than or equal to 18 mmHg when measured) and a P/F ratio of less than or equal to 200 mmHg. Acute lung injury (ALI) was also defined using the same criteria but with a P/F threshold of 300 mmHg; thus, ARDS was a subset of patients with ALI. Although this consensus definition better enabled comparative studies of epidemiology and mortality and enrollment in clinical trials, it was hampered by many limitations. Key among the limitations were the uncertainty of timing of the insult leading to ARDS, confusion surrounding the ALI category, ambiguity surrounding the use of P/F ratio relative to the application of PEEP, which may modify this ratio, marked inter-observer variation in the interpretation of chest radiography, and controversies in excluding volume overload or heart failure as the primary cause of respiratory failure. The current Berlin definition of ARDS addresses these limitations. It specifies an acute time frame for the development of ARDS (within 1 week of known clinical insult or new or worsening respiratory symptoms), stipulates minimum ventilator settings (PEEP of 5 cm H_2O or more), and clarifies chest radiography criteria as well as the adjudication of respiratory failure from volume overload or heart failure. Furthermore, the Berlin definition removes the ALI term and classifies ARDS into three categories (mild, moderate, and severe) to facilitate prognostication [11, 12].

Despite nearly five decades of study into ARDS, there are still no specific therapies beyond low tidal mechanical ventilation to reduce the mechanical stress placed on the injured lung. However, even with the advent of protective ventilation ARDS, mortality has not significantly declined below 40% [12, 13].

7.2 Epidemiology/Morbidity

Various studies have attempted to identify the incidence, outcomes, and population metrics of ARDS. But, the epidemiology of ARDS suffers from the lack of a true diagnostic test. Despite standardized definitions, most are hampered by inter-observer variability in ascertainment of cases, variations in validity of case definitions, geographic differences in availability of medical resources such as intensive care unit (ICU) beds, heterogeneity of risk factors among populations, and problems with determining mortality that can be directly attributed to ARDS, leading to inconsistencies of epidemiological measures [11].

The Large Observational Study to Understand the Global Impact of Severe Acute Respiratory Failure (LUNG-SAFE) is the latest cross-sectional study that provides data on the epidemiology of ARDS. Globally, ARDS accounts for 10% of intensive care unit admissions, representing more than three million patients with ARDS annually [11, 14]. Of the 12,906 patients who received mechanical ventilation, 23.4% fulfilled the Berlin definition of ARDS [11].

ARDS affects approximately 200,000 patients each year in the United States, resulting in nearly 75,000 deaths annually, more than breast cancer or HIV infection [15, 16]. Mortality from ARDS remains high, ranging from 35% to 46%, with higher mortality being associated with greater degrees of lung injury severity at onset. Survivors may have substantial and persistent physical, neuropsychiatric, and neurocognitive morbidity that has been associated with significantly impaired quality of life, as long as 5 years after the patient has recovered from ARDS.

7.3 Cause/Symptoms

ARDS is characterized by impaired oxygenation and bilateral infiltrates on a chest radiograph. It is caused by various conditions like pneumonia, burns, sepsis, trauma, acute pancreatitis, aspiration, toxic inhalation transfusion, and cardiopulmonary bypass surgery (Table 7.1) [1, 5, 6]. The clinical hallmarks are hypoxemia and bilateral radiographic opacities, associated with increased venous admixture, increased physiological dead space, and decreased lung compliance. The morphological hallmark of the acute phase is diffuse alveolar damage (i.e., edema, inflammation, hyaline membrane, or hemorrhage) [5].

A variety of clinical risk factors have been associated with the development of ARDS and fall into two broad categories: direct and indirect lung injury (Table 7.1).

Table 7.1 Direct and indirect etiological factors contributing to ARDS

S. No	Direct injury of the lung
1	Aspiration
2	Pneumonia
3	Inhalation injury
4	Drowning
5	Pulmonary contusion
S. No	Indirect injury of the lung
1	Sepsis
2	Trauma-induced injury/Shock
3	Severe burns
4	Pancreatitis
5	Cardiopulmonary bypass
6	Drug overdose
7	Head injury

Table 7.2 ARDS biomarkers [24]

Pathway	Biomarkers
Endothelial	Ang 1/2
	vWF
	VEGF
Epithelial	RAGE
	SP-D
	KGF
Coagulation and fibrinolysis	PAI-1
Inflammatory	IL-1Beta
	TNF-a
	IL-8
	IL-18
	IL-10
	sTNF-RI/II

The symptoms of ARDS are potentially underrecognized by clinicians. Early recognition and subsequent optimal treatment of patients with ARDS may be facilitated by usage of biomarkers. Several biomarkers have been examined with regard to their discriminatory ability for the diagnosis of ARDS (Table 7.2). Surfactant protein D (SP-D) has been proposed as such a candidate. Lung inflammation and injury affect the synthesis and secretion of SP-D from lung epithelial cells into the systematic circulation [17–19]. Infants and children are vulnerable to severe respiratory insult as compared to adults. Therefore, adult-based clinical definitions and parameters of ARDS are not applicable in pediatrics due to anatomic and physiologic differences. Pediatric acute lung injury consensus conference (PALICC), defined the first pediatric-focused characterization of ARDS. In pediatric ARDS, the oxygen index (OI) or oxygen saturation index defines the stratification of the severity of the disease based on the oxygen deficit [20–23].

7.4 Pathophysiology of ARDS

ARDS, a clinical syndrome of noncardiogenic pulmonary edema, is characterized by hypoxemia, radiographic infiltrates, decreased functional residual capacity, and decreased lung compliance [5, 23].

The most common pathophysiology of ARDS are the following:

1. *Disruption of pulmonary endothelial and alveolar epithelial integrity*
2. *Alveolar Epithelial injury and dysfunction*
3. *Disruption of Lung endothelial homeostasis*
4. *Inflammatory dysfunction*
5. *Surfactant dysfunction*
6. *Coagulation and fibrinolysis dysfunction*

7.4.1 Disruption of Pulmonary Endothelial and Alveolar Epithelial Integrity

Alveolar epithelial cells (AECs) collaboratively form a tight barrier between atmosphere and fluid-filled tissue to enable normal gas exchange. The tight junctions of AECs provide intercellular sealing and are integral to the maintenance of the AEC barrier integrity [25]. The alveolar epithelium is coated with a thin layer of alveolar wall liquid, which is necessary for dispersion of surfactant, transfer of gases, and host defense against inhaled pathogens. Integrity of this barrier is critical for gas exchange, and separation of the aqueous and gaseous compartments. Disruption and failure of reconstitution of the AEC barrier result in catastrophic consequences, leading to alveolar flooding with protein-rich edema fluid and subsequent devastating fibrotic scarring. Cytokines (interleukin-1 [IL-1], IL-8, tumor necrosis factor-a [TNF-a]) and lipid mediators (leukotriene B4) are attracted to alveoli and, in response to these proinflammatory mediators, neutrophils are recruited into the pulmonary interstitium and alveoli. The presence of protein, fibrinogen, and fibrin degradation products in the alveolar fluid results in surfactant degradation [6, 21, 22, 25].

7.4.2 Alveolar Epithelial Injury and Dysfunction

The alveolar wall is lined by two types of AECs: type I and type II AECs. The flat type I AECs and capillary endothelial cells constitute the blood–air barrier that facilitates efficient gas exchange. The cuboidal type II AECs secrete a surfactant that is believed to contribute to the lowering of alveolar surface tension. Apart from this, it is also responsible for the removal of excess alveolar fluid through sodium-dependent intracellular transport. Type II AECs proliferate and differentiate to Type I cells after injury.

Decreased alveolar fluid clearance is associated with severity and worse clinical outcomes and increased mortality in ARDS. Direct alveolar epithelial injury and indirect alveolar capillary injury (Table 7.1) cause barrier breakdown and inability of the alveolar epithelium to remove excess alveolar fluid. Surfactant protein D (SP-D), a marker of alveolar epithelial injury, has been proposed as a potentially useful biomarker for diagnosis of ARDS in a few studies [17] (Fig. 7.1).

7.4.3 Disruption of Lung Endothelial Homeostasis

Dysregulated endothelial activation and the resultant loss of homoeostatic mechanisms are aspects of ARDS pathobiology [6, 26]. Pulmonary endothelium is a dynamic, metabolically active organ that modulates several key regulatory functions including leucocyte diapedesis, intravascular coagulation, vasomotor tone, and solute and fluid trafficking via regulation of barrier permeability. Reactive oxygen species (ROS) and reactive nitrogen species production by activated cells saturate local antioxidants and contribute to tissue injury directly via downregulation of VE-cadherin, upregulation of neutrophil adhesion molecule expression, and release of neutrophil chemotactic factors. Endothelial-specific proteins, such as von Willebrand factor and angiotensin-converting enzyme activity, correlate with ARDS mortality. Moreover, activated endothelial cells also assume a procoagulant phenotype by increasing the expression of platelet adhesion molecules, intra-alveolar and intravascular fibrin deposition, and release of activators of the extrinsic coagulation cascade [1, 26–28].

7.4.4 Inflammatory Dysfunction

Several studies have demonstrated evidence for dysregulation of inflammatory pathways in ARDS and their association with outcome. There is a strong correlation between mortality and upregulated levels of proinflammatory (IL-6, IL-8, IL-18, MIP-1b, TNF-a) and anti-inflammatory cytokines (IL-1RA, IL-10, and TNF-R2). These cytokines were associated with ARDS illness severity, including the P/F ratio, OI, pediatric risk of mortality score (PRISM-3), ICU morbidity, and biochemical evidence of endothelial injury, including elevated plasma angiopoietin 2 and soluble thrombomodulin [4, 6, 29].

When alveolar macrophages are activated, they recruit neutrophils and circulating macrophages to the alveoli. Neutrophils communicate between the vessel wall and platelets, which results in endothelial injury and releases neutrophil extracellular traps, which may also cause damage to the lung [30, 31].

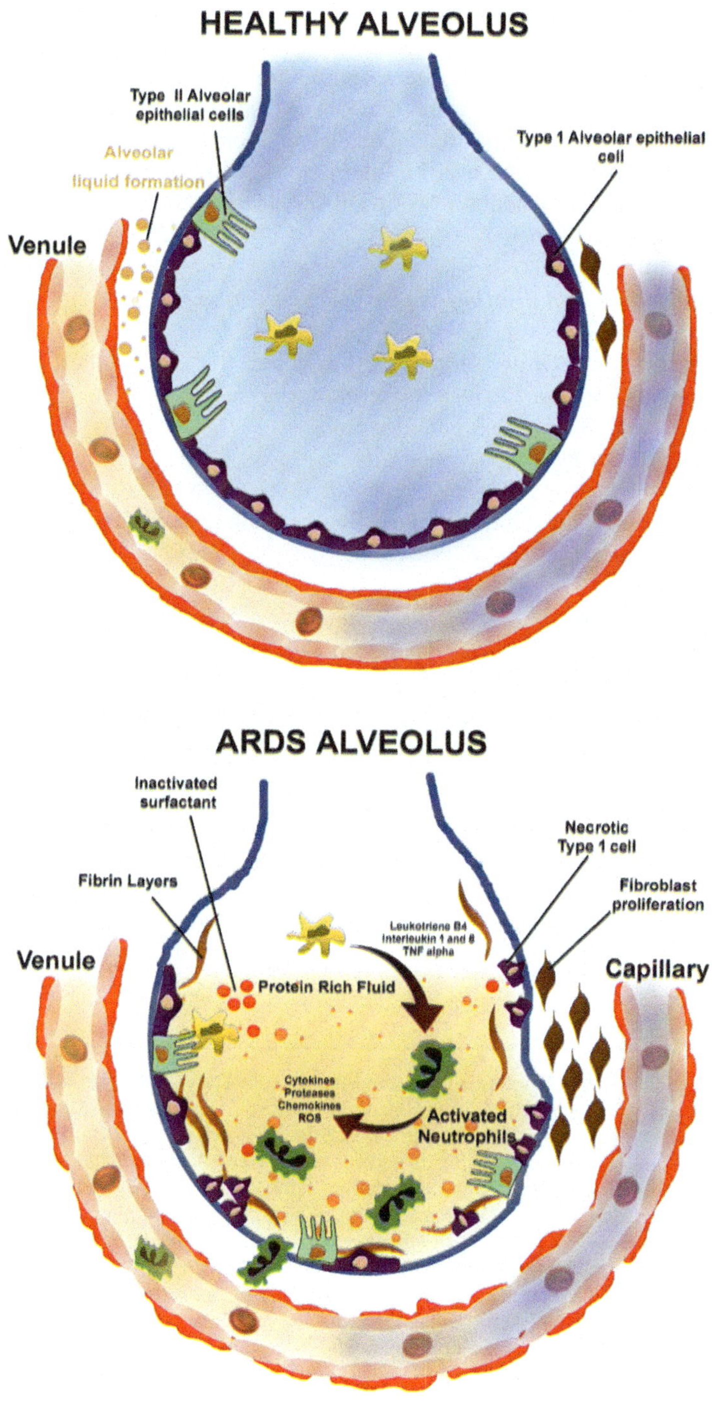

Fig. 7.1 Schematic representation of healthy alveolus and pathophysiology in ARDS: In the healthy alveolus (**Top**), the alveolar epithelium and capillary endothelium are intact, which

7.5 Current Therapies for ARDS

Despite decades of research, treatment options for ARDS are limited. Supportive care with mechanical ventilation remains the mainstay of management [32]. Most advances in ARDS therapeutics have been through changes in mechanical ventilation methods, culminating in a 2017 International Clinical Practice Guideline for mechanical ventilation on adults with ARDS [14, 15, 24, 32]. The guidelines address six interventions:

1. *low tidal volume and inspiratory pressure ventilation*
2. *prone positioning*
3. *high-frequency oscillatory ventilation*
4. *higher versus lower positive end-expiratory pressure*
5. *lung recruitment maneuvers and*
6. *extracorporeal membrane oxygenation*

Most of the current treatment is supportive and palliative, with no current disease-modifying therapies available [24].

7.5.1 Management-Based Therapy for ARDS

A standard therapy for ARDS is mainly based and reliant on management of pulmonary dysfunction; however, the identification involves non-pulmonary organ dysfunction also.

7.5.1.1 Treatment of the Inciting Clinical Disorder

ARDS is an outcome of several disease processes, which mainly include trauma, ischemia reperfusion, pneumonia, multiple transfusions, sepsis, and aspiration of gastric contents [33, 34]. Several of these have a direct treatment based on

---

Fig. 7.1 (continued) maintains the air-filled, fluid-free alveoli. The alveolar wall liquid formation is required for gas exchange, which is the medium for dispersal of the surfactant and alveolar macrophages, thereby maintaining alveolar stability and host defenses. (**Bottom**) In contrast, the alveolar space in ARDS looks highly disturbed with severe flooding with solutes and large molecules such as albumin. This fluid accumulation is due to the loss of epithelial and endothelial barrier integrity, leading to severe pulmonary edema. The endothelium of pulmonary micro-vessels gets activated; there is high influx of proinflammatory mediators. This leads to the recruitment of leukocytes into the pulmonary interstitium and alveoli. There are also high amounts of fibrin deposition due to increased concentration of fibrinogen and fibrin degradation products in the edema fluid. Depletion of surfactant leads to increase in surface tension and loss of alveolar shape and integrity. There is also fibroblast proliferation, ROS generation, and NET (neutrophil extracellular traps) in the diseased alveoli

antibiotics/antimicrobials, which however needs a careful examination for the type of pathogen involved in inciting the disease such as bacteria (Mycoplasma or Legionella) or fungi (Pneumocystis carinii). Sometimes ALI/ARDS is incited by extrapulmonary infections, e.g., urinary tract, pulmonary infection, or biliary tract infection, which hence warrants a thorough clinical examination. The clinical treatment should take the clinical history of the patient into account. In some situations, like transfusions or gastric aspirations, stopping the recurrence is the optimal treatment method along with good supportive care [33–36].

7.5.1.2 Mechanical Ventilation

ARDS generates an alveolar dead space, an impaired pulmonary compliance. The required amount of breathing is too high a work for the voluntary pulmonary system, which may lead to a ventilatory failure pulmonary acidosis and hypercapnia [37]. Overall, there is a huge respiratory burden, which demands an extra support to be functional. In such situations, mechanical ventilation serves as a backbone to respiration and hence is an essential supplementary care. Mechanical ventilation not only acts as a mainstay of supportive care but also provides sufficient time for natural healing and drug treatments [36, 38].

7.5.1.3 Effective Oxygenation (PEEP and FIO2)

An ARDS patient needs effective oxygenation at the start of mechanical ventilation, which is a high priority measure. During mechanical ventilation, positive end-expiratory pressure (PEEP) and fraction of inspired oxygen (FiO2) provide effective oxygenation and support arterial oxygenation and hence are crucial. PEEP and FiO2 are associated with serious limitations, which can be avoided by keeping the FiO2/PEEP index in check. For human subjects, FiO2 $<50\%$ is considered safe [39–42]. PEEP improves arterial oxygenation and decreases intrapulmonary shunt. It keeps a check on FiO2 while allowing adequate arterial oxygenation [43, 44].

7.5.1.4 Vasodilators

ARDS patients are known to have modest pulmonary arterial hypertension, which has been demonstrated to progress with the progression of disease. The rise is a multifactorial process and can make the disease severe by affecting the vascular bed and hypoxic vasoconstriction or sometimes cardiac dysfunction. Several studies have attempted to reduce the pulmonary hypertension to evaluate its effect on progression of ARDS. There are reports of using hydralazine in animal models, which has proven effective though [36, 45]. Continuous infusion of prostaglandin E1 has proven effective in clinical cases also [46]. Nitric oxide (NO) is an effective endogenous vasodilator. Encouraged from promised results obtained in animal models, clinicians attempted to use gaseous NO to treat pulmonary hypertension in ARDS patients; however, mild and transient success in clinical cases of ARDS was noted [47–51].

7.5.1.5 Infection Management in ARDS

Uncontrolled infection is a prominent feature associated with ALI/ARDS. Often, lung infection becomes a causal factor for development of ALI/ARDS [51]. However, infection may occur as an outcome of ARDS development, though reports of non-pulmonary sepsis are also known to cause ARDS. There is a high amount of risk associated with development of pneumonia and catheter-related sepsis also known as nosocomial infections in patients receiving ventilation, which is an area of investigation that is being highly investigated for quite some time [36, 52, 53]. Administration of antibiotics/antimicrobials does not help always. Therefore, infections are managed by frequent washing of hands by medical personnel, nonstop suction of subglottic secretions to avoid their aspiration, and the usage of new endotracheal tubes to avoid making of a bacterial biofilm. Almost all the management strategies for nosocomial pneumonia in ARDS are contentious. One of the important aspects that adds to this is the ambiguity in the diagnosis itself. There is a significant overlap between ARDS diagnosis and clinical data obtained from pneumonia, as the immune cell infiltration is highly similar in both pathologies [54, 55].

7.5.2 Drawbacks of the Current Pharmacological Treatment

Despite several decades of investigation into potential treatment strategies, use of lung-protective ventilation remains the only proven therapy to decrease mortality in ARDS [2]. In patients with ARDS, recruitment maneuvers improve oxygenation, but this is a temporary approach that does not improve mortality. Clinical trials of β2-agonists, statins, surfactants, and keratinocyte growth factor (KGF) have been disappointing. In addition, monoclonal antibodies (anti-TNF) and TNFR fusion protein have also been unconvincing. Glucocorticoids may improve oxygenation and airway pressures in established ARDS, but have failed to demonstrate a role in preventive therapy. In patients with pneumonia, steroids may improve radiological appearances, but again does not improve mortality [24, 56]. Trials conducted on established ARDS investigated different doses and duration of treatment, preventing generalization of the results. However, analysis suggests that if steroids are started 14 days or more after the diagnosis of ARDS, they can be harmful. The combination of inhaled β2-agonists and glucocorticoid administered early in patients at risk of ARDS has recently shown to prevent development of ARDS and improve oxygenation but its effect on mortality has not been demonstrated [24].

Despite intense investigation, no specific pharmacological treatment for ARDS has been shown to affect the mortality, even though preclinical trials in animal models have looked promising. Therefore, targeting a single pathogenetic pathway is not unlikely to be advantageous due to the complexity of the mechanisms involved [24].

7.6 Future Directions in Therapeutics and Perspectives

No pharmacologic treatments aimed at the underlying pathology have been shown to be effective, and management remains supportive with lung-protective mechanical ventilation. Guidelines on mechanical ventilation in patients with acute respiratory distress syndrome can assist clinicians in delivering evidence-based interventions that may lead to improved outcomes [15].

Even after 50 years of study, ARDS still looks like a threatening enemy to defeat. Studies on ARDS incidence consistently show that the disease is not rare, albeit often not recognized by clinicians. ARDS is undertreated and basic ventilator strategies are not yet standardly optimized, despite major advances in the management of mechanical ventilation and non-ventilatory strategies, aimed at preventing the VILI. Although mortality associated with ARDS is decreasing in clinical trials, it remains unchanged at approximately 40% in major observational studies. Various factors contribute to the mortality associated with ARDS. They include patient age and illness severity, country-level socioeconomic status, ventilator management, and ICU organizational method. This suggests the need of a commonly accepted therapeutic strategy for ARDS, which should be the prerogative of all the countries including the less-developed ones [57, 58]. Molecular mechanisms identifying the susceptibility of injury and aberrant activation of alveolar epithelial cells and pulmonary endothelial cells would be pivotal in moving toward the positive outcomes of these intractable diseases.

The characterization of the ARDS sub-phenotype by blood biomarkers may help clinicians to select patients who may benefit from specific therapeutic strategies and ultimately tailor the treatment of our single patient. In fact, it has been proved that a high PEEP strategy in ARDS patients affected the major outcome only in the hyperinflammatory sub-phenotype. Moreover, the restrictive fluid strategy was beneficial in the same selected ARDS patients. More studies are needed to further explore the benefits of different therapies based on a particular ARDS biomarker profile [24, 59]. To further reduce mortality, the therapy of ARDS should possibly take genetic difference among patients and the origin of ARDS into account, such as the primary or the secondary ARDS.

In the future, by understanding the role of biomarkers in the pathophysiology of ARDS and lung injury, it is hoped that this will provide rational therapeutic targets and ultimately improve clinical care.

References

1. Ware LB, Matthay MA (2000) The acute respiratory distress syndrome. N Engl J Med 342:1334–1349
2. Alessandri F, Pugliese F, Ranieri VM (2018) The role of rescue therapies in the treatment of severe ARDS. Respir Care 63:92–101
3. Ashbaugh DG, Bigelow DB, Petty TL, Levine BE (1967) Acute respiratory distress in adults. Lancet 2:319–323

4. Roy GB, Lorraine BW, Yves B, Michael AM (2001) Treatment of ARDS. Chest 120:1347–1367
5. ARDS Definition Task Force, Ranieri VM, Rubenfeld GD et al (2012) Acute respiratory distress syndrome: the Berlin Definition. JAMA 307:2526–2533
6. Heidemann SM, Nair A, Bulut Y, Sapru A (2017) Pathophysiology and management of acute respiratory distress syndrome in children. Pediatr Clin North Am 64:1017–1037
7. Sapru A, Flori H, Quasney MW et al (2015) Pathobiology of acute respiratory distress syndrome. Pediatr Crit Care Med 16:S6–S22
8. Katz R (1987) Adult respiratory distress syndrome in children. Clin Chest Med 8:635–639
9. Sherrill DL, Camilli A, Lebowitz MD (1989) On the temporal relationships between lung function and somatic growth. Am Rev Respir Dis 140:638–644
10. Wang X, Dockery DW, Wypij D et al (1993) Pulmonary function between 6 and 18 years of age. Pediatr Pulmonol 15:75–88
11. Nanchal RS, Truwit JD (2018) Recent advances in understanding and treating acute respiratory distress syndrome. F1000Res 7:F1000 Faculty Rev-1322
12. Villar J, Sulemanji D, Kacmarek RM (2014) The acute respiratory distress syndrome: incidence and mortality, has it changed? Curr Opin Crit Care 20:3–9
13. Wang T, Gross C, Desai AA et al (2017) Endothelial cell signaling and ventilator-induced lung injury: molecular mechanisms, genomic analyses, and therapeutic targets. Am J Physiol Lung Cell Mol Physiol 312:L452–L476
14. Fan E, Brodie D, Slutsky AS (2018) Acute respiratory distress syndrome: advances in diagnosis and treatment. JAMA 319:698–710
15. Fan E, Del Sorbo L, Goligher EC, Hodgson CL, Munshi L, Walkey AJ, Adhikari NKJ, Amato MBP, Branson R, Brower RG et al (2017) An official American Thoracic Society/European Society of Intensive Care Medicine/Society of Critical Care Medicine clinical practice guideline: mechanical ventilation in adult patients with acute respiratory distress syndrome. Am J Respir Crit Care Med 195:1253–1263
16. Rubenfeld GD, Caldwell E, Peabody E et al (2005) Incidence and outcomes of acute lung injury. N Engl J Med 353:1685–1693
17. Park J, Pabon M, Choi AMK et al (2017) Plasma surfactant protein-D as a diagnostic biomarker for acute respiratory distress syndrome: validation in US and Korean cohorts. BMC Pulm Med 17:204
18. Terpstra ML, Aman J, van Nieuw Amerongen GP, Groeneveld AB (2014) Plasma biomarkers for acute respiratory distress syndrome: a systematic review and meta-analysis. Crit Care Med 42:691–700
19. Hermans C, Bernard A (1999) Lung epithelium-specific proteins: characteristics and potential applications as markers. Am J Respir Crit Care Med 159:646–678
20. Flori H, Glidden D, Rutherford G et al (2005) Pediatric acute lung injury: prospective evaluation of risk factors associated with mortality. Am J Respir Crit Care Med 171:995–1001
21. Yehya N, Servaes S, Thomas NJ (2015) Characterizing degree of lung injury in pediatric acute respiratory distress syndrome. Crit Care Med 43:937–946
22. Zimmerman JJ, Akhtar SR, Caldwell E et al (2009) Incidence and outcomes of pediatric acute lung injury. Pediatrics 124:87–95
23. Cheifetz IM (2016) Year in review 2015: pediatric ARDS. Respir Care 61:980–985
24. Spadaro S, Park M, Turrini C et al (2019) Biomarkers for Acute Respiratory Distress syndrome and prospects for personalised medicine. J Inflamm (Lond) 16:1
25. Yanagi S, Tsubouchi H, Miura A, Matsumoto N, Nakazato M (2015) Breakdown of epithelial barrier integrity and overdrive activation of alveolar epithelial cells in the pathogenesis of acute respiratory distress syndrome and lung fibrosis. Biomed Res Int 2015:573210
26. Bachofen M, Weibel ER (1977) Alterations of the gas exchange apparatus in adult respiratory insufficiency associated with septicemia. Am Rev Respir Dis 116:589–615
27. Ware LB, Eisner MD, Thompson BT et al (2004) Significance of von Willebrand factor in septic and nonseptic patients with acute lung injury. Am J Respir Crit Care Med 170:766–772

28. Orfanos SE, Armaganidis A, Glynos C et al (2000) Pulmonary capillary endothelium bound angiotensin-converting enzyme activity in acute lung injury. Circulation 102:2011–2018
29. Parsons PE, Eisner MD, Thompson BT et al (2005) Lower tidal volume ventilation and plasma cytokine markers of inflammation in patients with acute lung injury. Crit Care Med 33:1–2
30. Aggarwal NR, King LS, D'Alessio FR (2014) Diverse macrophage populations mediate acute lung inflammation and resolution. Am J Physiol Lung Cell Mol Physiol 306:L709–L725
31. Caudrillier A, Kessenbrock K, Gilliss BM et al (2012) Platelets induce neutrophil extracellular traps in transfusion-related acute lung injury. J Clin Invest 122:2661–2671
32. Fan E, Needham DM, Stewart TE (2005) Ventilatory management of acute lung injury and acute respiratory distress syndrome. JAMA 294:2889–2896
33. Anderson ID, Fearon KC, Grant IS (1996) Laparotomy for abdominal sepsis in the critically ill. Br J Surg 83:535–539
34. Sinanan M, Maier RV, Carrico CJ (1984) Laparotomy for intraabdominal sepsis in patients in an ICUs. Arch Surg 119:652–658
35. Doyle RL, Szaflarski N, Modin GW et al (1995) Identification of patients with acute lung injury: predictors of mortality. Am J Respir Crit Care Med 152:1818–1824
36. Brower RG, Ware LB, Berthiaume Y, Matthay MA (2001) Treatment of ARDS. Chest 120:1347–1367
37. Falke KJ, Pontoppidan H, Kumar A et al (1972) Ventilation with end-expiratory pressure in acute lung disease. J Clin Invest 51:2315–2323
38. Lamy M, Fallat RJ, Koeniger E et al (1976) Pathologic features and mechanisms of hypoxemia in adult respiratory distress syndrome. Am Rev Respir Dis 114:267–284
39. Royston BD, Webster NR, Nunn JF (1990) Time course of changes in lung permeability and edema in the rat exposed to 100% oxygen. J Appl Physiol 69:1532–1537
40. Fracica PJ, Knapp MJ, Piantadosi CA, Takeda K, Fulkerson WJ, Coleman RE, Wolfe WG, Crapo JD (1991) Responses of baboons to prolonged hyperoxia: physiology and qualitative pathology. J Appl Physiol 71:2352–2362
41. Royer F, Martin DJ, Benchetrit G, Grimbert FA (1988) Increase in pulmonary capillary permeability in dogs exposed to 100% O2. J Appl Physiol 65:1140–1146
42. Fox RB, Hoidal JR, Brown DM, Repine JE (1981) Pulmonary inflammation due to oxygen toxicity: involvement of chemotactic factors and polymorphonuclear leukocytes. Am Rev Respir Dis 123:521–523
43. Shank JC, Latshaw RF (1980) Adult respiratory distress syndrome. Am Fam Physician 21:107–114
44. Falke KJ, Pontoppidan H, Kumar A, Leith DE, Geffin B, Laver MB (1972) Ventilation with end-expiratory pressure in acute lung disease. J Clin Invest 51:2315–2323
45. Harrison WD, Raizen M, Ghignone M, Girling L, Slykerman LJ, Prewitt RM (1983) Treatment of canine low pressure pulmonary edema: nitroprusside versus hydralazine. Am Rev Respir Dis 128:857–861
46. Bone RC, Slotman G, Maunder R, Silverman H, Hyers TM, Kerstein MD, Ursprung JJ (1989) Randomized double-blind, multicenter study of prostaglandin E1 in patients with the adult respiratory distress syndrome: Prostaglandin E1 Study Group. Chest 96:114–119
47. Frostell C, Fratacci MD, Wain JC, Jones R, Zapol WM (1991) Inhaled nitric oxide: a selective pulmonary vasodilator reversing hypoxic pulmonary vasoconstriction. Circulation 83:2038–2047
48. Fratacci MD, Frostell CG, Chen TY, Wain JC Jr, Robinson DR, Zapol WM (1991) Inhaled nitric oxide: a selective pulmonary vasodilator of heparin-protamine vasoconstriction in sheep. Anesthesiology 75:990–999
49. Shah NS, Nakayama DK, Jacob TD (1994) Efficacy of inhaled nitric oxide in a porcine model of adult respiratory distress syndrome. Arch Surg 129:158–164
50. Rossaint R, Falke KJ, López F, Slama K, Pison U, Zapol WM (1993) Inhaled nitric oxide for the adult respiratory distress syndrome. N Engl J Med 328:399–405

51. Rayees S, Joshi JC, Tauseef M, Anwar M, Baweja S, Rochford I, Joshi B, Hollenberg MD, Reddy SP, Mehta D (2019) PAR2-mediated cAMP generation suppresses TRPV4-dependent Ca2+ signaling in alveolar macrophages to resolve TLR4-induced inflammation. Cell Rep 27:793–805
52. Sutherland KR, Maunder RJ, Milberg JA, Allen DL, Hudson LD (1995) Pulmonary infection during the acute respiratory distress syndrome. Am J Respir Crit Care Med 152:550–556
53. Meduri GU, Wunderink RG, Leeper KV Jr, Jones CB, Tolley E, Mayhall G (1994) Causes of fever and pulmonary densities in patients with clinical manifestations of ventilator-associated pneumonia. Chest 106:221–235
54. Seidenfeld JJ, Bell RC, Harris GD, Johanson WG Jr (1986) Incidence, site, and outcome of infections in patients with the adult respiratory distress syndrome. Am Rev Respir Dis 134:12–16
55. American Thoracic Society (1995) Hospital-acquired pneumonia in adults: diagnosis, assessment of severity, initial antimicrobial therapy, and preventative strategies; a consensus statement. Am J Respir Crit Care Med 153:1711–1725
56. Steinberg KP, Hudson LD, Goodman RB, Hough CL, Lanken PN, Hyzy R, Thompson BT, Ancukiewicz M (2006) National Heart L. Blood institute acute respiratory distress syndrome clinical trials N: efficacy and safety of corticosteroids for persistent acute respiratory distress syndrome. N Engl J Med 354:1671–1684
57. McNicholas BA, Rooney GM, Laffey JG (2018) Lessons to learn from epidemiologic studies in ARDS. Curr Opin Crit Care 24:41–48
58. Rezoagli E, Fumagalli R, Bellani G (2017) Definition and epidemiology of acute respiratory distress syndrome. Ann Transl Med 5:282
59. Calfee CS, Delucchi K, Parsons PE, Thompson BT, Ware LB, Matthay MA, Network NA (2014) Subphenotypes in acute respiratory distress syndrome: latent class analysis of data from two randomised controlled trials. Lancet Respir Med 2:611–620

Chronic Obstructive Pulmonary Disease: An Update on Therapeutics and Pathophysiological Understanding

8

Kaiser Jehan Peerzada

Abstract

Chronic obstructive pulmonary disease (COPD) is a common inflammatory disease of the airways, characterized by persistent respiratory symptoms and airflow limitations, and is significantly increasing in prevalence worldwide. It is the fourth leading cause of death in the developed world. COPD is likely to become the number two cause of death by the third decade of the twenty-first century if this increase in prevalence continues. The number of patients with COPD in fact may be greater than statistics indicate, since typically, the disease is not diagnosed until the patient presents with a first exacerbation. The pathological indicators of COPD are bronchitis (inflammation of the small airways) and emphysema (destruction of lung parenchyma). The most important clinical and functional consequences of these abnormalities are exacerbations and airflow limitations. There is a complex interaction between airway abnormalities and emphysema that leads to the development of airflow limitation, causing airway narrowing and debilitating bouts of shortness of breath, wheezing, chest tightness, and cough.

Keywords

COPD · Emphysema · Airways inflammation · COPD epidemiology · Spirometry · Management of COPD · Treatment strategies

K. Jehan Peerzada (✉)
Pharmacology Division, Indian Institute of Integrative Medicine (CSIR), Jammu Tawi, India
e-mail: kaiserpeerzada@gmail.com

S. Rayees et al. (eds.), *Chronic Lung Diseases*,
https://doi.org/10.1007/978-981-15-3734-9_8

8.1 Introduction

Chronic obstructive pulmonary disease (COPD) is a severe and a chronic inflammatory disease, which affects over 170 million people and accounts for over three million deaths each year globally [1, 2]. The prevalence has increased, at least in part, due to an increasing cigarette consumption in developing countries and the overall longer survival rate [3, 4]. Although to a greater extent, exposure to cigarette smoke is the prime identifiable cause of COPD, additionally, exposure to certain occupational dusts and chemicals (grain, isocyanates, cadmium, coal, welding fumes), exposures to smoke and fuel used for cooking and heating at homes, and a genetic predisposition (primarily α_1-antitrypsin deficiency) have been associated with the disease [5, 6].

COPD patients often experience persistent respiratory symptoms like dyspnea (shortness of breath), and are also vulnerable to episodic COPD exacerbations (an acute worsening of respiratory symptoms), which are triggered by various factors such as air pollution and infections, and as a result, the adjacent alveoli and vasculature are affected [7]. Uncontrolled COPD exacerbations often cause an irreversible loss in lung function and/or complications requiring medical attention [8]. Symptoms range from chronic productive cough to exhausting dyspnea [9]. COPD remains a major burden on patients, their caregivers, and the health-care system. It is the eighth ranked cause of disability as measured by disability-adjusted life years (DALYs) [10]. An understanding of this disorder dates back centuries [11] including recognition of the components of emphysema and chronic bronchitic [12, 13]. The diagnostic approach to this disorder was revolutionized with the invention of the spirometer [14] and timed measurement of forced exhalation of expired air [15–17].

8.2 Epidemiology

According to the latest estimates from Global Burden of Disease study published in *The Lancet Respiratory Medicine* journal, there has been a huge impact of the two most common chronic respiratory diseases, COPD and asthma, globally, with 3.2 million deaths and about 0.4 million deaths respectively, caused by these diseases, in 2015. According to this study, asthma is the most common chronic respiratory disease worldwide, with twice the number of cases of COPD in 2015, but surprisingly, the deaths from COPD have been reported to be eight times more common than deaths from asthma [10]. Many cases of COPD can be treated or prevented with affordable interventions, but people are often left undiagnosed, misdiagnosed, or undertreated. The only fundamental tool used to define, point, and survey population prevalence is spirometry [18, 19]. Under the sponsorship of the Burden of Obstructive Lung Disease (BOLD) initiative, surveys have been done in 29 countries, and are still in progress in additional nine countries [20]. Further, population estimates are being provided by other two initiatives conducted in five Colombian cities (PREPOCOL) [21] and in five Latin American capital cities,

Proyecto LatinoAmericano de Investigacion en Obstruccion Pulmonar (PLATINO) [22]. In order to define COPD, there is still no universal consensus about the thresholds of spirometry findings, in spite of using comparable methods [23]. The two dominant case definitions for airflow limitation compatible with COPD are a value of less than 0.70 for the ratio of forced expiratory volume (FEV1) to forced vital capacity (FVC), or the lower limit of normal (LLN) method of deriving a threshold as the fifth percentile of FEV1:FVC in a healthy control population [19]. Again, no universal LLN threshold exists, as it is presumed to vary between populations [24], since most people singled out for COPD based on spirometry findings report not having been diagnosed prior to survey [25]. Nevertheless, to quantify COPD and its severity, the international initiatives such as PREPOCOL (Prevalencia de EPOC en Colombia), PLATINO, BOLD (Burden of Obstructive lung diseases), and EPI-SCAN (The Epidemiologic Study of COPD in Spain) have used standardized population spirometry. However, their estimations are still biased due to an absence of consensus on case definitions and other sources of measurement. The examination by PLATINO, conducted in persons greater than 40 years, from each of five Latin American countries—Brazil, Chile, Mexico, Uruguay, and Venezuela—showed that the prevalence of COPD increased steeply with age, with the highest prevalence among those >60 years. They showed that prevalence in the total population ranged from a low of 7.8% in Mexico, to a high of 19.7% in Montevideo, Uruguay [26, 27].

COPD is ranked among the top 20 conditions causing disability globally, and stands at rank eighth as a cause of disease burden, according to the baseline projections made in the Global Burden of Disease Study (GBDS) as a measure for disability-adjusted life years (DALYs) [10]. The DALYs for a specific condition are the sum of years lost because of premature mortality and years of life lived with disability, adjusted for the severity of disability. The GBD Study found that COPD is an increasing contributor to disability and mortality globally. Yet, the measurement of mortality, prevalence, and other population indicators of this disease is complicated due to improper categorization and an absence of concord about case definitions. The prevalence and the death rates have been seen to increase sharply with age [10].

The largest increase in the smoking-related mortality is estimated to occur in China, India, and other Asian countries [28]. Most of the available data on the disease are reported from the Western world, but still it is being equally recognized from Asia and Africa. Unlike Europe and the United States, the Asian continent is far reaching and diversified with pronounced variance in social and health-care infrastructure in different countries. While some of the countries have very high capital, the others are either impoverished or in different stages of economic development. These components probably can affect the disease prevalence significantly. COPD interestingly is a problem of great magnitude in almost all these countries. Therefore, an epidemic of chronic respiratory disability is genuinely feared taking into account a large population of the world residing in these regions [29]. Work place exposures to chemical agents, fumes, and dust (organic and inorganic) are undoubtedly an underrated risk factor for COPD [30]. According to National Health and Nutrition

Examination Survey III, based on US population of about 10,000 adults between age 30 and 75 years, the fraction of COPD attributable to workplace exposures was estimated to be 19.2% [31], which is consistent with the statement published by the American Thoracic Society that occupational exposures account for 10–20% of respiratory diseases either symptomatically or by impairing functionality [32]. Burning of wood, coal, animal dung, and crop residues, generally burned in poorly ventilated rooms, open fires or poorly functioning stoves, may also lead to high levels of indoor air pollution, thereby increasing the risk factor for COPD [33]. There is a substantial population risk worldwide since almost three billion people use coal and biomass as their main source of energy for their household needs [34]. Similarly, there is high prevalence of COPD among nonsmoking women due to use of biomass fuels for cooking, in parts of the Middle East, Africa, and Asia [35, 36]. Indoor air pollution resulting from the burning of wood and other biomass fuels is estimated to kill two million women and children each year [37].

One systematic review and meta-analysis, including studies carried out in 28 countries between 1990 and 2004, provided evidence that the prevalence of COPD is appreciably higher in smokers and ex-smokers compared to nonsmokers, in those $\geq$40 years of age compared to those <40 [38]. With the increasing prevalence of smoking and aging populations in developing countries, the prevalence of COPD is expected to rise over the next decade and by 2030, there may be over 4.5 million deaths annually from COPD and related conditions [39, 40].

Although cigarette smoking is the most well-studied risk factor, it is not the only risk factor for COPD, and there is consistent evidence from epidemiologic studies that nonsmokers may also develop chronic airflow limitation [41]. Nevertheless, nonsmokers with chronic airflow limitation have fewer symptoms, milder disease, and lower burden of systemic inflammation and they appear to have a low risk of lung cancer, or cardiovascular comorbidities, compared to smokers with COPD, though there are reports that they may have an increased risk of pneumonia and mortality from respiratory failure [42]. Morbidity from COPD may be affected by other associated chronic conditions that are related to smoking and aging (e.g., cardiovascular diseases or musculoskeletal impairment) [43], which might interfere with COPD management and significantly impair patient's health status, in addition to being drivers for hospitalizations and affect cost of treatments [44]. There may be an underestimation of the burden of COPD under areas that rely on administrative health data, particularly those that only record hospitalizations [45]. Also, the reliability on mortality data to be recorded as COPD-related deaths is problematic. Although COPD is often a primary cause of death, it is more likely to be listed as a contributory cause of death or omitted from the death certificate entirely [19]. However, it is clear that COPD is one of the most important causes of death in most countries.

8.2.1 Economic Burden

COPD is associated with significant economic burden. Subsequently, with larger number of cases, more people have been reported to be living with disability, with the highest burden of disability from people residing in developing regions. In 2015, disease burden due to COPD was reported to be highest in Papua New Guinea, India, Lesotho, and Nepal, and lowest in some countries in high-income Asia Pacific, Central Europe, North Africa, and the Middle East, the Caribbean, Western Europe, and Andean Latin America [10]. India can be projected as a classical example with reference to the rising burden of chronic diseases. In an estimate in 2005, the burden from chronic respiratory disease was shown to account for 7% of deaths and 3% of DALYs lost diseases, out of 53% of all deaths and 44% of DALYs lost, and from other chronic diseases [46]. This was obviously an underassessment since there was inadequate information available on COPD. Information now available on COPD from India is bound to tremendously expand this burden [47–49]. It is estimated that, on an average, an Indian COPD patient spends about 15% of his income on smoking products and up to 30% on disease management. Reports from several other Asian countries are equally alarming [50]. In the European Union, the total direct costs of respiratory diseases have been reported to be approximately 6% of their total health-care budget, with COPD accounting for 56% (38.6 billion Euros) of the cost of respiratory disease [51], while the estimated direct and indirect costs of COPD are $32.0 billion and $20.4 billion respectively, in the USA [52].

A significant proportion of the total burden of COPD in the health-care system is accounted by exacerbations, as there is a significant direct relationship between the severity of the disease and the cost of care as the disease progresses. For example, with disease severity, the charges for hospitalization and roving oxygen costs rise. The economic value of the care provided by family members to people with COPD is disregarded; therefore, any estimate of expenditure for home-based care is marginalized. Since the healthcare sector does not provide long-term supportive care services for severely disabled individuals, COPD may force at least two individuals to leave the workplace—the affected individual and a family member who must now stay home to care for their disabled relative [53]. The indirect costs of COPD may represent a serious threat to the economy since human capital is one of the most important national assets for developing a nation. Interestingly, it has been seen that the causes for COPD have opposite patterns according to the geographic areas. In high- and middle-income countries, tobacco smoke is the biggest risk factor; meanwhile, in low-income countries, exposure to indoor air pollution, such as the use of biomass fuels for cooking and heating, causes the COPD burden [54].

8.3 Symptoms and Causes of the Disease

The most common symptoms of COPD are breathlessness, or a "need for air," and a chronic productive cough [55]. However, COPD is not just simply a "smoker's cough," but an underdiagnosed, life-threatening lung disease that may progressively lead to death. Inhaled air containing irritants start cascade of inflammation in the airways [56]. Inflammation of the large airways does not contribute directly to the decrease in airflow characteristic of COPD. There is a conclusive relation between and the amount of damage to the small airways and the progression of impairment as a disease, which probably points that the inflammation found there is a major contributor to functional deterioration [57].

Airflow limitation related to COPD is thus believed to be due to a combination of small airway disease and emphysema, which together lead to chronic inflammation in patients. Ultimately, it leads to fibrosis of the airway and proliferation of smooth muscle owing to persistently amplified muscle tone. Eventually, airway narrowing is severe enough to result in limitation of airflow leading to a decrease in functionality [58].

8.4 Pathophysiology of COPD

Pathophysiology describes the changes that a disease or condition causes in a person's physical function as it develops. There has been significant progress in the pathological description and pathophysiological analysis of COPD in the twenty-first century. There is a blockage in the airways of a COPD patient since the site of airflow obstruction is located there only. The structural abnormalities are peribronchiolar and characterized by deposition of extra cellular material consisting of thick fibers of collagen [59], and by luminal obstruction by mucous exudates, a typical feature of the small airways in COPD patients [60]. This peribronchiolar fibrosis is an important determinant of airway obstruction and a significant contributor to the bronchiolar wall thickening [61].

In COPD, lung function is reduced as the airways and air sacs are damaged. Normally, during inhalation, air travels down bronchial tubes, which branch into thinner millennial channels called bronchioles, and reaches the tiny air sacs or alveoli. There are more than 300 million alveoli in the lungs. Once air makes its way to the air sacs, oxygen passes through the walls of the air sac into the capillaries that surround them and at the same time, carbon dioxide moves from the capillaries into the air sacs. These events happen simultaneously and are referred to as gas exchange. Air sacs are elastic and during the process of "breathing in," they are inflated with air like a balloon. The air sacs deflate during the "breathing out" process. Energy is utilized to blow the air sacs up.

People with COPD have airflow limitations, either due to the loss of elasticity of the airways and air sacs, or because the walls between the air sacs are partially or completely damaged [58]. There can be an airway inflammation, causing thickening of walls or a hyper production of mucus, causing the airways to be plugged. Together or independently, these manifest into conditions like emphysema, chronic bronchitis, refractory asthma, or a combination of all. Each one of them leads to a different problem with the airways and sacs. The ultimate effect is limitation of airflow, with a forced expiratory volume in 1 s (FEV1): forced vital capacity (FVC) ratio less than 70% of the predicted value, being the criteria for diagnosis according to the Global Initiative for Chronic Obstructive Lung Disease (GOLD) grading system [62].

8.4.1 Emphysema

It represents the destruction of the lung parenchyma without obvious fibrosis. The damage to the air sacs in the lungs causes them to lose their plasticity and trap the air instead, resulting in difficulty to expel all air from the lungs, thereby affecting the lung efficiency [63]. This leads to the air trapping and causes the lungs to hyper inflate. With excessive air in the lungs, breathing takes additional efforts, contributing to shortness of breath and even extreme fatigue.

8.4.2 Chronic Bronchitis

Bronchitis is an inflammation of the small airways that causes narrowing of the lumen and an active constriction. It results from an increase in airways inflammation and mucus production, leading to the airways lining being constantly irritated and inflamed. With the result, the cilia that helps to move the mucus along the airways to be removed from lungs by coughing also loses its function or even disappears altogether [64]. Overall inflammation causes narrowing of the airways, making breathing more difficult.

8.4.3 Refractory Asthma

The main difference between asthma and COPD is that asthmatic condition is reversible and COPD is an irreversible one [65]. In refractory asthma, a patient does not respond to asthma medications. Asthma presents in attacks that cause the airways to become more tight and swollen. People with refractory asthma cannot revert the airways to their natural state using medications [64].

8.5 Biology of Disease

The inflammation of airways caused by infiltration of neutrophils is a hallmark of COPD [66]. Inhalation of noxious substances irritates the lining of the respiratory tract and causes macrophage activation. These macrophages travel to the lungs where they undergo phagocytosis and release neutrophil chemotactic factors, including IL-8 and leukotriene B_4 (LTB_4). Macrophage activation leads to recruitment of additional macrophages through the action of various chemokines. Recruitment of neutrophils and their activation lead to secretion of several serine proteases including neutrophil elastase (NE), matrix metalloproteinase (MMP), as well as myeloperoxidase (MPO) all of which contribute to destruction of connective tissues in the lung parenchyma [67]. The whole process concludes in the development of emphysema and the increased mucus secretion common to patients with COPD [68]. Many studies have reported an increase in MMPs in plasma and bronchoalveolar lavage fluid (BALF) of emphysematic patients, and seen to increase airways obstruction by destroying structural components of extra cellular matrix (ECM) [69, 70]. Inflammatory cells release oxidants that are capable of directly damaging the lung structure. Many studies have implicated the importance of inflammatory cells in COPD, which is characterized by increased numbers of CD8-positive T-lymphocytes, neutrophils, macrophages and B-lymphocytes [71, 72]. However, currently little is known about the role of the individual cell types that infiltrate the lungs in COPD.

In emphysema, there is an abnormal permanent enlargement of air spaces beyond the terminal bronchioles, accompanied by destruction of their walls without obvious fibrosis, the mechanism of which is probably multifactorial and not much elucidated. The physiological repair of epithelial gaps caused by epithelial aggression (tobacco smoke) is mediated by the plasticity of the lung epithelium by the process of trans-differentiation [73]. In trans-differentiation, one type of differentiated cell transforms into another type of differentiated cell, which is distinct from the usual differentiation process in which undifferentiated progenitor cells (e.g., stem cells and basal epithelial cells) give rise to differentiated cells (e.g. ciliated cells, goblet cells, and Clara cells) [74]. The condition in emphysema is believed to be related to imbalance of protease–protease inhibitor, and also to mechanisms involving apoptosis, senescence, and autoimmunity, since deformity in epithelial and/or endothelial alveolar cell survival programs has been observed. An imbalance between proliferation and apoptosis could thus account for the pathogenesis of emphysema. It has been suggested that the inception of this imbalances is followed by an increased apoptosis, cellular senescence phenomena, and autoimmunity [73].

The advent of moderate emphysema with drop in respiratory function is also associated with the normal pulmonary aging, and is called senile emphysema [75]. In pneumocytes and pulmonary endothelial cells of emphysematous smoking patients, an overexpression of telomere shortening and p16 (markers of senescence) has been reported [76]. Tobacco smoke has been seen to induce senescence in normal pulmonary culture fibroblasts, while as fibroblasts of emphysematous lungs were seen to proliferate less than those of controls [77–79].

Alveolar destruction may also promote abundant apoptosis, which might be incited by three distinct pathways involving caspases: (1) The extrinsic pathway (receptor-mediated) induced by soluble mediators like TNF-alpha and sFasL (soluble Fas ligand or CD95L), (2) the intrinsic pathway induced by physicochemical stress or deprivation of growth factors, and (3) the endoplasmic pathway induced by hypoxia [80]. In animals, emphysema may be induced by inhibition of the *vascular endothelial growth factor* (VEGF) pathway and its receptors [81, 82], or by the administration of active caspases [83]. Compared to control, an increase in apoptosis in alveolar epithelial and/or endothelial cells of COPD patients has been reported [84]. In the lung tissue of severe COPD patients, an induction of caspase-3 has been observed [85], while Galectin-3, which is an inhibitor of apoptosis in leukocytes and epithelial cells, has also been reported to be increased significantly in the bronchioles of such patients, correlated with an increased proliferation of bronchiolar epithelium [86].

An implication of an autoimmune disorder has been suggested in the pathogenesis of emphysema, which is coupled to either an immune response to microbial antigens causing a cross-reaction against self-antigens (molecular mimicry), or by a polyclonal activation of B-lymphocytes due to defective removal of dead cells [87]. The first evidence of autoimmunity in COPD in an animal model has been reported by Taraseviciene-Stewart et al. [88]. Lee et al. also have shown that emphysema in humans is associated with the development of anti-elastin autoimmunity correlated with the severity of the disease [89]. Studies show that the development of emphysema in animal models and in humans is accompanied by an autoimmune reaction against the epithelium and/or alveolar endothelium, but it is not clear whether autoimmunity is a cause of emphysema, or emphysema leads to autoimmunity [89, 90]. In the evolution and development of COPD, pulmonary vascular abnormalities have been an important component. They can cause changes in gas exchange [91] or show up in a serious complication of COPD in the form of pulmonary arterial hypertension [92]. Endothelial cells play a crucial role in the regulation of vascular tone and therefore in the adaptation of pulmonary vascular resistance to changes in blood flow. Early endothelial dysfunction seen in COPD leads to changes in the regulation and release of certain vasodilators neuromediators such as NO or prostacyclin or vasoconstrictors such as endothelin-1 or angiotensin [93]. A decline in the expression of NO synthase in the pulmonary arteries has been seen in smokers, which is significantly lower in the more severe COPD patients [94].

The integrity of the airways in response to external agents such as smoke is maintained by an innate immune and perhaps adaptive response, characterized by the recruitment of inflammatory cells into the airways. Therefore, inflammation of the airway is constant during COPD and affects the proximal as well as distal airways [95]. A pathological study of distal airways has indicated that with an increase in the severity of bronchial obstruction, there is a significant rise of infiltration of macrophages, neutrophils, $CD4^+$ and $CD8^+$ T cells, and B-lymphocytes [72–75, 96, 97].

Alveolar infiltration of macrophages has long been described in patients with COPD [97] and these macrophages may have a peculiar phenotypic characteristic. Studies show that about 46% of the macrophages taken from induced sputum of COPD subjects are smaller, compared to 7% in healthy subjects. These smaller macrophages have a proinflammatory phenotype and overexpress CD14 and HLA-DR, and also show an increased secretion of TNF-alpha, both before and after stimulation with bacterial lipopolysaccharide [98].

Others have reported that macrophages from BAL fluid in COPD patients express less CD86 and CD11a, which are costimulatory and adhesion molecules respectively, compared to healthy smokers [99].

The presence of neutrophils in the bronchoalveolar lavage (BAL) fluid in patients with COPD has been identified in many studies [100]. An increase in neutrophil recruitment was identified in the 1980s, highlighting the potential role of proteases secreted by these cells in the degradation of matrix proteins, and the pathogenesis of emphysema [101]. Additionally, neutrophils may trigger secretion of mucus by the bronchiolar epithelium [102, 103].

The number of dendritic cells in bronchioles has been reported to increase with the severity of bronchial obstruction in COPD patients. Dendritic cells, which are the main antigen-presenting cells in the airways, have been shown to be increased in expression of CD1a in BAL fluid of smokers. CD1a represents immature dendritic cells [104–106]. In the alveolar walls of emphysematous patients, an increase in $CD4^+$ and $CD8^+$ T cells has been observed [107]. Numerous other studies have also confirmed the increase in $CD8^+$ cells in the BAL fluid of COPD patients compared to smokers without bronchial obstruction [108, 109].

Mast cells have been less frequently explored in studies of COPD pathology, despite several indications of their possible involvement. Mast cells play a central role in allergic and inflammatory reactions and a significant contribution of mediators released from mast cells occurs in allergic indications.

These cells, discovered in 1878, are highly specialized exocytic cells that line the surfaces of the body, including the skin, the respiratory tract, and the gastrointestinal tract [110]. They are in prime position to react to foreign particles such as pollen and bacteria by interfacing with the external environment. They have primarily been regarded as effector cells promoting IgE-mediated allergic reactions following secondary exposure to allergens [111, 112].

It is now known that mast cells participate more diversely in both allergy and infection, and also seem to play a critical role in exacerbations of allergic disease and in the setting of infection. Therefore, by increasing the understanding of the role of mast cells in innate and adaptive immunity to infectious pathogens, we may be able to discover better treatments to prevent development of allergic disease and exacerbations of established disease, since in allergen sensitization, COPD exacerbations and infection control, the pathways and mechanisms involved are probably unvaried [113]. It has been reported that in smokers, there is an increase in numbers of mast cells in the airway epithelium [114], and increased levels of the mast cell products, histamine and tryptase, have also been detected in BAL fluid [115] and tryptase-positive cells are almost invariably mast cells [113].

8.6 Current Treatments and Their Drawbacks

The mechanisms involved in COPD are much less well understood than are those of asthma, which results in slow outcome of research aimed at improving treatment for COPD. Additionally, COPD is generally misinterpreted as being untreatable because of difficulty in reversing airway obstruction. Owing to its link to smoking, COPD sometimes is considered a result of the patient's own accountability. Smoking abstinence has the greatest capacity to influence the natural history of COPD, and is in fact the only intervention identified till date that decelerates the progression of the disease. If effective resources and time are dedicated to smoking cessation, long-term quit success rates of up to 25% can be achieved [9]. Along with individual approaches, legislative smoking bans are also effective in increasing quit rates and reducing damage from second-hand smoke exposure [116]. Counseling delivered by physicians and other health professionals significantly increases quit rates over self-initiated strategies. Even brief (3-min) periods of advice urging a smoker to quit have been reported to improve smoking cessation rates [117, 118]. A few nicotine replacement products have been put up as pharmacotherapies for smoking cessation, which include nicotine gum, inhaler, nasal sprays, transdermal patch, sublingual tablet, or lozenges. These have been shown to reliably increase long-term smoking abstinence rates significantly [119, 120]. However, medical contraindications reported for nicotine replacement therapy like myocardial infarction or stroke render them unsafe as sole replacements [121, 122]. Continuous chewing of nicotine gum produces secretions that are swallowed rather than absorbed through the buccal mucosa, resulting in little or no absorption, and potentially causing nausea. The efficacy of E-cigarettes as a form of nicotine replacement therapy happens to be controversial.

By definition, COPD patients have restriction of airflow that is usually gradual and significant, but not altogether irreversible. Essentially, COPD is progression in the rate of functional decline of the lungs caused by the inhalation of proinflammatory particles. Early strategies for the treatment of COPD are in many respects significantly different from current recommendations. Initially, the number of pharmacologic agents available to treat COPD was limited. The primary agents given for the treatment were antibiotics, mucolytics, and nonselective sympathomimetics (sometimes prescribed with a sedative to counter balance hostile effects). Antibiotics have been approached and administered routinely to treat patients with COPD, since decades. The administration of these agents is a necessary component of the treatment of infection associated with COPD, but since patients with chronic bronchitis have high susceptibility to pulmonary infections than other patients without COPD, antibiotic therapy must be used more judiciously today than it was in the past. With steady increase in prevalence of antibiotic resistance, patients today are screened more carefully for antibiotic need. Those patients who are younger and without other severe underlying medical problems or frequent exacerbations are less likely in requirement of broad-spectrum antibiotic therapy [123, 124]. Routine use is now discouraged.

Mucolytic drugs (carbocysteine and *N*-acetylcysteine (NAC)) are thought to increase the expectoration of sputum by reducing its density. However, the usefulness of these agents for most patients with COPD has been called into question [125]. Simply decreasing the viscosity of mucus may be unproductive without an overall decrease in the quantity of secretions. Data regarding the use of *N*-acetylcysteine, the most widely studied of the mucolytic agents, are conflicting. No data exist to demonstrate an improvement in lung function with mucolytic therapy [126, 127]. The previous GOLD report surmises that regular use of mucolytic agents, such as NAC and carbocysteine, reduces the risk of exacerbation if used in appropriate patients [128].

Use of indiscriminate sympathomimetic agents (ephedrine, epinephrine) for treatment, which was once a fairly common practice, has mostly been replaced now by selective β_2-agonists, which are widely used and recommended in current treatment guidelines [129]. Despite having been recognized for a long time as a cheap and effective therapy for the treatment of COPD, theophylline is downgraded to third-line therapy in the treatment of airway diseases due to its relatively low efficacy and frequent side effects (cardiovascular effects) [130, 131]. Because theophylline has a narrow therapeutic range, a relatively high number of potentially interacting drugs, and high-risk toxic symptoms (such as seizures and arrhythmias), treatment with theophylline has become unpopular in many parts of the world [132].

8.7 Treatment Strategies

Bronchodilators are medications that increase FEV1 and/or change other spirometric variables. The mode of action of bronchodilators is manifested by alterations in the tone of airway smooth muscle, which leads to improvements in expiratory flow. These processes consider distension of the airways and tend to reduce hyperinflation rather than change elastic recoil in lungs [133].

Drugs in this component of treatment comprise short-acting (albuterol, levalbuterol, and salbutamol) and long-acting (salmeterol, formoterol) beta 2-agonists, anticholinergics (ipratropium, tiotropium), and to a lesser extent theophylline. These drugs are prescribed either alone or in combination as required to maintain symptom control, and are most often advised on a regular basis to prevent or reduce symptoms. However, since toxicity is dose-related, use of short-acting bronchodilators on a regular basis is not generally recommended.

8.7.1 Beta2-Agonists

The principal action of beta2-agonists is to relax airway smooth muscle. These act by increased cyclic AMP via stimulation of beta2-adrenergic receptors so that functional antagonism to bronchoconstriction is produced. There are short-acting (SABA) and long-acting (LABA) beta2-agonists. The effect of SABAs usually wears off within 4–6 h [134, 135].

Requisite and regular use of SABAs improves FEV1 and symptoms [136]. In spite of a large collection of beneficial data available for short-acting β_2-agonists, approximately one-third of patients show insignificant response in lung function tests after using these agents. LABAs show duration of action of 12 or more hours. Formoterol and salmeterol have been shown to significantly improve FEV1, lung volumes, dyspnea, health status, exacerbation rate, and reduced number of hospitalizations, but have no effect on mortality and lung function decline [137, 138]. At currently recommended doses, β_2-agonists do not reach their maximum bronchodilatory potential, and with increase in dose, the abundance of adverse effects increases as well (tremor and reflex tachycardia), which is troublesome in some older patients. With higher doses, tachyphylaxis is reckoned to occur [139].

8.7.2 Antimuscarinic Drugs

Anticholinergics or antimuscarinic drugs block the bronchoconstrictor effects of acetylcholine on M3 muscarinic receptors expressed in airway smooth muscle. There are short-acting [SAMA] (ipratropium and oxitropium) and long-acting antimuscarinics [LAMA] (tiotropium, aclidinium, and glycopyrronium bromide), which have sustained binding to M2 and M3 muscarinic receptors, respectively, thereby prolonging the duration of bronchodilator effect [140]. It has been concluded from a random control review that ipratropium alone provided small benefits over short-acting beta2-agonist in terms of lung function, requirement for oral steroids and health status. Tiotropium also has been shown to improve symptoms and health status by improving the effectiveness of pulmonary rehabilitation and reduced exacerbations and other related hospitalizations [141]. The main side effect, however, is dryness of mouth [142]. Some patients have reported a bitter, metallic taste with use of ipratropium, and with regular treatment of ipratropium bromide, a small increase in cardiovascular events in patients are reported [143, 144].

8.7.3 Methylxanthines

The effects of xanthine derivatives (theophylline and doxofylline) in COPD are controversial, as they act either as nonselective phosphodiesterase inhibitors or as bronchodilators. Theophylline is a weak, nonselective inhibitor of phosphodiesterase (PDE) isoenzymes, and it antagonizes adenosine A1 and A2 receptors, and exhibits a broad spectrum of anti-inflammatory effects by increasing interleukin-10. Theophylline is metabolized by cytochrome P450 enzymes and its clearance declines with age [145]. Doxofylline, on the other hand, exhibits both bronchodilator and antiinflammatory activity [146].

8.7.4 Corticosteroids

Long-term therapy with systemic corticosteroids has no place in the management of stable COPD, as it contributes to increased morbidity in the form of intercostal myopathy [147]. Inhaled corticosteroids (ICS), though frequently prescribed for patients with COPD, are similarly not recommended for maintenance therapy for most patients. Because of the uncertainty regarding dose–response relationships and long-term safety, recommendations are only to prescribe inhaled corticosteroids in long-term in patients who demonstrate a definite spirometric response identifiable within 3 months, or if a patient has an FEV1 below 50% of predicted value in addition to repeated exacerbations requiring antibiotic therapy or oral steroids [148]. It has been established that regular treatment with ICS alone does not modify the mortality or long-term decline of FEV1 in patients with COPD. In vivo data suggest that the dose–response relationships and long-term (>3 years) safety of inhaled corticosteroids (ICS) in patients with COPD are unclear and require further investigation [149, 150].

8.7.5 Combination Therapy

Combining bronchodilators with other mechanistic drugs with different durations of action has been seen to increase the degree of bronchodilation with a lower risk of side effects compared to increasing the dose of a single bronchodilator [151]. Combinations of short-acting beta agonists with short-acting muscarinic antagonist have presented better results in improving FEV1 and symptoms, compared to monotherapy [152]. Inhalers in the form of combination of formoterol and tiotropium have shown a significant impact on FEV1 than either component alone [153]. There are other diverse combinations of a LABA and LAMA available as inhalers, which have been reported to improve lung function compared to placebo. An ICS combined with a LABA has been seen to be more effective than ICS alone in improving lung function, health status, and reducing exacerbations in patients with moderate-to-very severe COPD [154, 155].

8.7.5.1 Triple Inhaled Therapy

This advancement in combination of inhalers as LABA, LAMA, and ICS (triple therapy) is achieved by various approaches and has been reported to improve lung function in COPD patients [156–158].

8.7.6 Oral Glucocorticoids

One of the debilitating side effects of oral glucocorticoids is steroid myopathy, which can contribute to muscle weakness, decreased functionality, and respiratory failure in subjects with very severe COPD [147]. Therefore, their role in the chronic daily is limited because of a lack of overall benefit against a high rate of systemic complications.

8.7.7 Alpha-1 Antitrypsin Augmentation Therapy

The rational strategy to manage the development and progression of lung disease in alpha 1 antitrypsin deficient (AATD) patients is alpha-1-antitrypsin augmentation [159]. Because AATD is rare, formal clinical trials to assess efficacy with conventional spirometric outcome have never been undertaken. Additionally, the main limitation for this therapy is very high cost and lack of availability in many countries [160].

8.8 Future Directions in Therapeutics

Despite there being extensive data in understanding of the complex disease processes of COPD, no current therapy till date is sufficiently effective to treat and reverse the underlying process of inflammation and functional decline. To reduce the disease progression and the mortality of COPD patients, effective antiinflammatory treatments are required. The factors that contribute to the etiology of this complex disease process are versatile and include both genetic and environmental factors. Cigarette smoking is the most important recognizable risk factor for COPD; however, the disease develops only in a minority of long-term smokers, suggesting that genetic factors contribute to the development of this disease. Therefore, it is critical to understand genes and their final product (proteins) in order to solve the underlying pathophysiological mechanism of the disease. But genetic assay through RNA quantification does not necessarily correlate with gene products, and further variations in protein expression are caused by posttranslational modification. Since the biological function is exhibited by the protein product, the most important step in the gene expression happens at the level of protein synthesis. New therapeutic approaches for COPD patients have been recommended through recent advances in the research on the underlying inflammation [161], which include new antioxidants, antagonists of cytokines or chemokines, inflammasome inhibitors, antiproteases, inhibitors for pro-inflammatory kinase, and agents that would reverse steroid resistance, and epigenetic modulation, some of which are undergoing clinical trials. In order to achieve the best management of disease, importance of accomplishment of complete pathophysiological evaluation and characterization of COPD patients is advised for selection of an appropriate treatment for each clinical phenotype. Therefore, further investigations for better understanding of the biological and pathophysiological processes of COPD are needed to achieve the goal of COPD management. Due to the heterogeneity of the disease and lack of an appropriate animal models and biomarkers for predicting therapeutic response, current understanding of the underlying disease mechanism is hampered, and is further impeded because of long-duration trials needed for demonstration of clinical efficacy. In order to understand the etiology of inflammatory diseases, recently, there has been a wide range of interest in using the proteomic approach to define disease markers and to identify the diagnostic options, and is now regarded as a powerful tool to identify novel diagnostic, prognostic, and therapeutic markers. The core element of the classical proteome research combines the multidimensional separation of proteins by 2-dimensional gel electrophoresis (2GE) or by multidimensional liquid chromatography (LC) or matrix assisted laser desorption/ionisation-time of flight (MALDI-TOF) [162].

The airways and particularly the alveoli are covered with a thin layer of epithelium lining fluid (ELF). This ELF is a rich source of many different cells and soluble components of the lungs and is imparted with significant functions of protecting the lung from undue aggressions and preserving its gas-exchange capacity. Therefore, the protein composition of the EFL is a reflection of effects of the external factors that hit the lungs and is of primary importance in the early diagnosis of a disease. It also has a role in the assessment and the characterization of lung disorders as well as in the search for disease markers. Numerous chemical, physical, and biological exposures, and finally lung diseases induce biochemical modifications of this ELF. The oldest and the most common means used up to now to get the samples of ELF that most accurately reflects its global protein composition is the bronchoalveolar lavage fluid (BALF). Analysis of BALF is most commonly employed to determine the protein composition of pulmonary airways. BALF contains cells (alveolar macrophages, lymphocytes, neutrophils, eosinophils, sometimes squamous epithelial cells, broncho epithelial cells, basophils, and mast cells) and a wide variety of soluble components (lipids, nucleic acids, and proteins/peptides) originating from ELF [163]. The study of BALF through proteomics helps to analyze thousands of proteins and thus provides comprehensive BALF proteome information that is essential toward understanding the molecular mechanisms underlying the lung inflammatory disease like COPD [164]. Therefore, protein profiling using the technique of 2DE and MALDI-TOF will help in the understanding of possible targets for inflammation and bronchoconstriction of COPD, which could be related to clinical benefit.

Recently, 2GE and multidimensional liquid chromatographic approaches have probably dominated the clinical proteomics field. However, new integrated and multidisciplinary approaches are still needed to increase the sensitivity of current proteomic analyses [165, 166]. Possibly, an integrative system biology approach based on the use of bioinformatics tools for data mining and integration, could allow building networks of proteins for identifying pathogenetic pathways of COPD [167, 168].

8.9 Perspective

Irrespective of magnificent progress in research, there are still large gaps in our understanding of the phenotypic heterogeneity of the lung diseases. This lack of knowledge resource applies even in the regulation of underlying mechanisms involved and functional significance of the diseases of the airways.

The number of patients with COPD has taken a lead. Some therapeutic strategies, once used routinely, are no longer considered appropriate. However, improvements to therapeutic approaches are being made, but still a substantial amount of research needs to be conducted to discover new modules of therapy and perhaps develop the agents that can slow down or halt the progressive functional decline of lungs. Based on the mechanisms of inflammation in COPD as we understand them, several areas for targeted therapy need to be studied. The disease markers to identify and validate the clinical efficacy of new agents are still underway. Efforts to define such markers need to be made to facilitate the advancement of COPD therapy. Additional studies are needed to examine the long-term effects of this therapy in patients receiving currently recommended COPD maintenance therapy.

References

1. Sana A, Somda SMA, Meda N, Bouland C (2018) Chronic obstructive pulmonary disease associated with biomass fuel use in women: a systematic review and meta-analysis. BMJ Open Respir Res 5(1):e000246
2. Global Burden of Disease Study Collaborators (2015) Global, regional, and national age-sex specific all-cause and cause-specific mortality for 240 causes of death, 1990-2013: a systematic analysis for the Global Burden of Disease Study 2013. Lancet 385(9963):117–171
3. Barnes PJ (2002) New treatments for COPD. Nat Rev Drug Discov 1:437–446
4. Prince MJ, Wu F, Guo Y, Gutierrez Robledo LM, O'Donnell M, Sullivan R, Yusuf S (2015) The burden of disease in older people and implications for health policy and practice. Lancet 385(9967):549–562
5. Pauwels RA, Buist AS, Ma P, Jenkins CR, Hurd SS, GOLD Scientific Committee (2001) Global strategy for the diagnosis, management and prevention of chronic obstructive pulmonary disease. National Heart, Lung, and Blood Institute/World Health Organization workshop report. Respir Care 46(8):798–825
6. Antó JM, Vermeire P, Vestbo J, Sunyer J (2001) Epidemiology of chronic obstructive pulmonary disease. Eur Respir J 17:982–994
7. Lowe KE, Regan EA, Anzueto A et al (2019) COPDGene 2019: redefining the diagnosis of chronic obstructive pulmonary disease. Chronic Obstr Pulm Dis 6(5):384–399
8. Shah SA, Velardo C, Farmer A, Tarassenko L (2017) Exacerbations in chronic obstructive pulmonary disease: identification and prediction using a digital health system. J Med Internet Res 19(3):e69
9. Yamada M, Ichinose M (2015) Cutting edge of COPD therapy: current pharmacological therapy and future direction. COPD Res Pract 1:5
10. Chronic Respiratory Disease Collaborators (2017) Global, regional, and national deaths, prevalence, disability-adjusted life years, and years lived with disability for chronic obstructive pulmonary disease and asthma, 1990-2015: a systematic analysis for the Global Burden of Disease Study 2015. Lancet Respir Med 5:691–706
11. Petty TL (2006) The history of COPD. Int J Chron Obstruct Pulmon Dis 1(1):3–14
12. Forbes J. Preface and notes. In: Laennec RTH. A treatise on the disease of the chest (English translation from the French). London: T and G Underwood;1821.
13. Badham C (1814) An essay on bronchitis: with a supplement containing remarks on simple pulmonary abscess, 2nd edn. J Callow, London
14. Hutchinson J (1846) On the capacity of the lungs, and on the respiratory functions, with a view of establishing a precise and easy method of detecting disease by the spirometer. Med Chir Trans 29:137–161
15. Tiffenau R, Pinelli AF (1947) Air curlant et air captive dans l'exploration de la function ventilatrice pulmonaire. Paris Med 133:624–628
16. Gaensler EA (1950) Air velocity index: a numerical expression of the functionally effective portion of ventilation. Am Rev Tuberc 62(1-A):17–28
17. Gaensler EA (1951) Analysis of the ventilatory defect by timed capacity measurements. Am Rev Tuberc 64:256–278
18. Rayees S, Malik F, Bukhari SI, Singh G (2014) Linking GATA-3 and interleukin-13: implications in asthma. Inflamm Res 63(4):255–265
19. Vogelmeier CF, Criner GJ, Martinez FJ et al (2017) Global strategy for the diagnosis, management, and prevention of chronic obstructive lung disease 2017 report: GOLD executive summary. Eur Respir J 49:1750214
20. BOLD-COPD International Research platform. http://www.boldstudy.org/index.html. Accessed 7 Feb 2017
21. Caballero A, Torres-Duque CA, Jaramillo C et al (2008) Prevalence of COPD in five Colombian cities situated at low, medium, and high altitude (PREPOCOL study). Chest 133:343–349

22. Menezes AMB, Victora CG, Perez-Padilla R, PLATINO Team (2004) The Platino project: methodology of a multicenter prevalence survey of chronic obstructive pulmonary disease in major Latin American cities. BMC Med Res Methodol 4:15
23. Vollmer WM, Gíslason T, Burney P et al (2009) Comparison of spirometry criteria for the diagnosis of COPD: results from the BOLD study. Eur Respir J 34:588–597
24. Quanjer PH, Stanojevic S, Cole TJ et al (2012) Multi-ethnic reference values for spirometry for the 3–95-yr age range: the global lung function 2012 equations. Eur Respir J 40:1324–1343
25. Lamprecht B, Soriano JB, Studnicka M et al (2015) Determinants of underdiagnosis of COPD in national and international surveys. Chest 148:971–985
26. Menezes AM, Perez-Padilla R, Jardim JR et al (2005) Chronic obstructive pulmonary disease in five Latin American cities (the PLATINO study): a prevalence study. Lancet 366 (9500):1875–1881
27. Menezes AM, Wehrmeister FC, Perez-Padilla R, Viana KP, Soares C, Müllerova H, Valdivia G, Jardim JR, Montes de Oca M (2017) The PLATINO study: description of the distribution, stability, and mortality according to the Global Initiative for Chronic Obstructive Lung Disease classification from 2007 to 2017. Int J COPD 12:1491–1501
28. Murray CJL, Lopez AD (1997) Alternative projection of mortality and disability by cause 1990-2020: global burden of disease study. Lancet 349:1498–1504
29. Yang JJ, Yu D, Wen W et al (2019) Tobacco smoking and mortality in Asia: a pooled meta-analysis. JAMA Netw Open 2(3):e191474
30. Paulin LM, Diette GB, Blanc PD, Putcha N, Eisner MD, Kanner RE, Belli AJ, Christenson S, Tashkin DP, Han M et al (2015) SPIROMICS Research Group. Occupational exposures are associated with worse morbidity in patients with chronic obstructive pulmonary disease. Am J Respir Crit Care Med 191:557–565
31. Abdool-Gaffar MS, Calligaro G, Wong ML, Smith C, Lalloo UG, Koegelenberg CFN, Dheda K, Allwood BW, Goolam-Mahomed A, van Zyl-Smit RN (2019) Management of chronic obstructive pulmonary disease—a position statement of the South African Thoracic Society: 2019 update. J Thorac Dis 11(11):4408–4427
32. Mahmood T, Singh RK, Kant S, Shukla AD, Chandra A, Srivastava RK (2017) Prevalence and etiological profile of chronic obstructive pulmonary disease in non-smokers. Lung India 34(2):122–126
33. Gan WQ, FitzGerald JM, Carlsten C, Sadatsafavi M, Brauer M (2013) Associations of ambient air pollution with chronic obstructive pulmonary disease hospitalization and mortality. Am J Respir Crit Care Med 187:721–727
34. Rajendra KC, Shukla SD, Gautam SS, Hansbro PM, O'Toole RF (2018) The role of environmental exposure to non-cigarette smoke in lung disease. Clin Transl Med 7:39
35. Tageldin MA, Nafti S, Khan JA, Nejjari C, Beji M, Mahboub B, Obeidat NM, Uzaslan E, Sayineri A, Wali S, Rashid N, Hasnaoui AE, BREATHE Study Group (2012) Distribution of COPD-related symptoms in the Middle East and North Africa: Results of the BREATHE study. Respir Med 106(S2):S25–S32
36. World health organization. https://www.who.int/respiratory/copd/causes/en/
37. Gordon SB, Bruce NG, Grigg J et al (2014) Respiratory risks from household air pollution in low- and middle-income countries. Lancet Respir Med 2:823–860
38. Bai JW, Chen XX, Liu S, Yu L, Xu JF (2017) Smoking cessation affects the natural history of COPD. Int J Chron Obstruct Pulmon Dis 12:3323–3328
39. Lopez AD, Shibuya K, Rao C et al (2006) Chronic obstructive pulmonary disease: current burden and future projections. Eur Respir J 27(2):397–412. 28
40. World Health Organization. Projections of mortality and causes of death, 2015 and 2030. http://www.who.int/healthinfo/global_burden_disease/projections/en/. Accessed 11 Sep 2016
41. Vogelmeier CF, Criner GJ, Martinez FJ, Anzueto A, Barnes PJ, Bourbeau J, Celli BR, Chen R, Decramer M, Fabbri LM, Frith P, Halpin DMG, López Varela MV, Nishimura M, Roche N, Rodriguez-Roisin R, Sin DD, Singh D, Stockley R, Vestbo J, Wedzicha JA, Agustí A (2017)

Global strategy for the diagnosis, management, and prevention of chronic obstructive lung disease 2017 report. GOLD executive summary. Am J Respir Crit Care Med 195(5):557–582
42. Thomsen M, Nordestgaard BG, Vestbo J, Lange P (2013) Characteristics and outcomes of chronic obstructive pulmonary disease in never smokers in Denmark: a prospective population study. Lancet Respir Med 1:543–550
43. Chen W, Thomas J, Sadatsafavi M, FitzGerald JM (2015) Risk of cardiovascular comorbidity in patients with chronic obstructive pulmonary disease: a systematic review and meta-analysis. Lancet Respir Med 3(8):631–639
44. Mannino DM, Higuchi K, Yu TC et al (2015) Economic burden of COPD in the presence of comorbidities. Chest 148(1):138–150
45. Stein BD, Bautista A, Schumock GT et al (2012) The validity of International Classification of Diseases, Ninth Revision, Clinical Modification diagnosis codes for identifying patients hospitalized for COPD exacerbations. Chest 141(1):87–93
46. Reddy KS, Shah B, Varghese C, Ramadoss A (2005) Responding to the threat of chronic diseases in India. Lancet 366:1744–1749
47. Jindal SK, Aggarwal AN, Gupta D (2001) A review of population studies from India to estimate national burden of chronic obstructive pulmonary disease and its association with smoking. Indian J Chest Dis Allied Sci 43:139–147
48. Ray D, Abel R, Selvaraj KG (1995) A 5-year prospective epidemiological study of chronic obstructive pulmonary disease in rural south India. Indian J Med Res 101:238–244
49. Jindal SK, Aggarwal AN, Chaudhry K, Chhabra SK, D'Souza GA, Gupta D et al (2006) Asthma Epidemiology Study Group. A multicentric study on epidemiology of chronic obstructive pulmonary disease and its relationship with tobacco smoking and environmental tobacco smoke exposure. Indian J Chest Dis Allied Sci 48:23–27
50. Jindal SK, Jindal SK (2006) Emergence of chronic obstructive pulmonary disease as an epidemic in India. Indian J Med Res 124:619–630
51. American Thoracic Society Foundation (2014) The global burden of lung disease. http://foundation.thoracic.org/news/global-burden.php. Accessed 28 Jul 2016
52. Guarascio AJ, Ray SM, Finch CK, Self TH (2013) The clinical and economic burden of chronic obstructive pulmonary disease in the USA. Clin Econ Outcom Res CEOR 5:235–245
53. Sin DD, Stafinski T, Ng YC, Bell NR, Jacobs P (2002) The impact of chronic obstructive pulmonary disease on work loss in the United States. Am J Respir Crit Care Med 165 (5):704–707
54. World Health Organisation (2016) Chronic obstructive pulmonary disease (COPD). http://www.who.int/mediacentre/factsheets/fs315/en/. Accessed 15 Jun 2017
55. Global Initiative for Chronic Obstructive Lung Disease (GOLD) (2014) Global strategy for the diagnosis, management and prevention of COPD. Available from http://www.goldcopd.org
56. Barnes PJ (2016) Inflammatory mechanisms in patients with chronic obstructive pulmonary disease. J Allergy Clin Immunol 138:16–27
57. Piqueras MG, Cosio MG (2001) Disease of the airways in chronic obstructive pulmonary disease. Eur Respir J 18(Suppl 34):S41–S49
58. Barnes PJ (2019) Small airway fibrosis in COPD. Int J Biochem Cell Biol 116:1–5
59. Wright JL, Postma DS, Kerstjens HA et al (2007) Airway remodeling in the smoke exposed guinea pig model. Inhal Toxicol 19:915–923
60. Koo H, Vasilescu DM, Booth S, Hsieh A, Katsamenis OL, Fishbane N, Elliott WM, Kirby M, Lackie PM, Sinclair I, Warner JA, Cooper JD, Coxson HO, Pare PD, Hogg JC, Hackett TL (2018) Small airways disease in mild and moderate chronic obstructive pulmonary disease: a cross-sectional study. Lancet Respir Med 6:591–602
61. Burgel PR, Bourdin A, Pilette C, Garcia G, Chanez P, Tillie-Leblond I (2013) Structural changes and inflammation in COPD: importance of distal airways. Structural abnormalities and inflammation in COPD: a focus on small airways. Respir Dis Rev 28:749–760

62. Vestbo J, Hurd SS, Agustí AG et al (2013) Global strategy for the diagnosis, management, and prevention of chronic obstructive pulmonary disease: GOLD executive summary. Am J Respir Crit Care Med 187:347–3652
63. Basbaum C, Jany B (1990) Plasticity in the airway epithelium. Am J Physiol 259:L38–L46
64. What happens to the lungs in COPD? Medically reviewed by Elaine K. Luo on September 30, 2019—written by Brian Wu. https://www.medicalnewstoday.com/articles/315687.php
65. Reilly JJ, Silverman EK, Shapiro SD (2015) Harrisons textbook of internal medicine, vol 2, 19th edn. McGraw Hill Professional, New York, NY, p 1700. Chapter 314
66. Wang Y, Jia M, Yan X et al (2017) Increased neutrophil gelatinase-associated lipocalin (NGAL) promotes airway remodelling in chronic obstructive pulmonary disease. Clin Sci 131(11):1147–1159
67. Bardoel BW, Kenny EF, Sollberger G, Zychlinsky A (2014) The balancing act of neutrophils. Cell Host Microbe 15(5):526–536
68. Tian P, Wen FQ (2015) Clinical significance of airway mucus hypersecretion in chronic obstructive pulmonary disease. J Transl Int Med 3(3):89–92
69. D'Armiento JM, Goldklang MP, Hardigan AA et al (2013) Increased matrix metalloproteinase (MMPs) levels do not predict disease severity or progression in emphysema. PLoS One 8(2): e56352
70. Ostridge K, Williams N, Kim V et al (2016) Relationship between pulmonary matrix metalloproteinases and quantitative CT markers of small airways disease and emphysema in COPD. Thorax 71(2):126–132
71. Wang Y, Xu J, Meng Y, Adcock IM, Yao X (2018) Role of inflammatory cells in airway remodeling in COPD. Int J Chron Obstruct Pulmon Dis 13:3341–3348
72. Polverino F, Seys LJ, Bracke KR, Owen CA (2016) B cells in chronic obstructive pulmonary disease: moving to center stage. Am J Physiol Lung Cell Mol Physiol 311(4):L687–L695
73. Burgel PR, Bourdin A, Pilette C, Garcia G, Chanez P, Tillie-Leblond I (2011) Structural abnormalities and inflammation in COPD: a focus on small airways. Res Dis Rev 28 (6):749–760
74. Avila PC (2011) Plasticity of airway epithelial cells. J Allergy Clin Immunol 128 (6):1225–1226
75. Mercado N, Ito K, Barnes PJ (2015) Emphysema could also be promoted by early senescence of alveolar cells, characterized by a decrease proliferation capacities and protein synthesis. Thorax 70:482–489
76. Tsuji T, Aoshiba K, Nagai A (2006) Alveolar cell senescence in patients with pulmonary emphysema. Am J Respir Crit Care Med 174:886–893
77. Holz O, Zuhlke I, Jaksztat E et al (2004) Lung fibroblasts from patients with emphysema show a reduced proliferation rate in culture. Eur Respir J 24:575–579
78. Nyunoya T, Monick MM, Klingelhutz A et al (2006) Cigarette smoke induces cellular senescence. Am J Respir Cell Mol Biol 35:681–688
79. Hikichi M, Mizumura K, Maruoka S, Gon Y (2019) Pathogenesis of chronic obstructive pulmonary disease (COPD) induced by cigarette smoke. J Thorac Dis 11(17):S2129–S2140
80. Aoshiba K, Yokohori N, Nagai A (2003) Alveolar wall apoptosis causes lung destruction and emphysematous changes. Am J Respir Cell Mol Biol 28:555–562
81. Kasahara Y, Tuder RM, Taraseviciene-Stewart L et al (2000) Inhibition of VEGF receptors causes lung cell apoptosis and emphysema. J Clin Invest 106:1311–1319
82. Tuder RM, Zhen L, Cho CY et al (2003) Oxidative stress and apoptosis interact and cause emphysema due to vascular endothelial growth factor receptor blockade. Am J Respir Cell Mol Biol 29:88–97
83. Kitaguchi Y, Taraseviciene-Stewart L, Hanaoka M, Natarajan R, Kraskauskas D, Voelkel NF (2012) Acrolein induces endoplasmic reticulum stress and causes airspace enlargement. PLoS One 7(5):e38038

84. Long Y, Liu X, Chen S et al (2018) miR-34a is involved in CSE-induced apoptosis of human pulmonary microvascular endothelial cells by targeting Notch-1 receptor protein. Respir Res 19(1):21–29
85. Sun X, Feng X, Zheng D, Li A, Li C, Li S, Zhao Z (2019) Ergosterol attenuates cigarette smoke extract-induced COPD by modulating inflammation, oxidative stress and apoptosis in vitro and in vivo. Clin Sci (Lond) 133(13):1523–1536
86. Pilette C, Colinet B, Kiss R et al (2007) Increased galectin-3 expression and intra-epithelial neutrophils in small airways in severe COPD. Eur Respir J 29:914–922
87. Davidson A, Diamond B (2001) Autoimmune diseases. N Engl J Med 345:340–350
88. Taraseviciene-Stewart L, Scerbavicius R, Choe KH et al (2005) An animal model of autoimmune emphysema. Am J Respir Crit Care Med 171:734–742
89. Lee SH, Goswami S, Grudo A et al (2007) Antielastin autoimmunity in tobacco smoking-induced emphysema. Nat Med 13:567–569
90. Feghali-Bostwick CA, Gadgil AS, Otterbein LE et al (2008) Autoantibodies in patients with chronic obstructive pulmonary disease. Am J Respir Crit Care Med 177:156–163
91. Magee F, Wright JL, Wiggs BR et al (1988) Pulmonary vascular structure and function in chronic obstructive pulmonary disease. Thorax 43:183–189
92. Barbera JA, Peinado VI, Santos S (2003) Pulmonary hypertension in chronic obstructive pulmonary disease. Eur Respir J 21:892–905
93. Peinado VI, Barbera JA, Ramirez J et al (1998) Endothelial dysfunction in pulmonary arteries of patients with mild COPD. Am J Physiol 274:L908–L913
94. Barbera JA, Peinado VI, Santos S et al (2001) Reduced expression of endothelial nitric oxide synthase in pulmonary arteries of smokers. Am J Respir Crit Care Med 164:709–713
95. Barnes PJ (2017) Cellular and molecular mechanisms of asthma and COPD. Clin Sci (Lond) 131(13):1541–1558
96. Mizutani N, Nabe T, Yoshino S (2014) IL-17A promotes the exacerbation of IL-33-induced airway hyperresponsiveness by enhancing neutrophilic inflammation via CXCR2 signaling in mice. J Immunol 192(4):1372–1384
97. Finkelstein R, Ma HD, Ghezzo H et al (1995) Morphometry of small airways in smokers and its relationship to emphysema type and hyperresponsiveness. Am J Respir Crit Care Med 152:267–276
98. Frankenberger M, Menzel M, Betz R et al (2004) Characterization of a population of small macrophages in induced sputum of patients with chronic obstructive pulmonary disease and healthy volunteers. Clin Exp Immunol 138:507–516
99. Lofdahl JM, Wahlstrom J, Skold CM (2006) Different inflammatory cell pattern and macrophage phenotype in chronic obstructive pulmonary disease patients, smokers and non-smokers. Clin Exp Immunol 145:428–437
100. Hartjes FJ, Vonk JM, Faiz A, Hiemstra PS, Lapperre TS, Kerstjens HAM, Postma DS, van den Berge M (2018) Predictive value of eosinophils and neutrophils on clinical effects of ICS in COPD. Respirology 23(11):1023–1031
101. Senior RM, Griffin GL, Mecham RP (1980) Chemotactic activity of elastin-derived peptides. J Clin Invest 66(4):859–862
102. Park JW, Shin NR, Shin IS, Kwon OK, Kim JS, Oh SR, Kim JH, Ahn KS (2016) Silibinin inhibits neutrophilic inflammation and mucus secretion induced by cigarette smoke via suppression of ERK-SP1 pathway. Phytother Res 30(12):1926–1936
103. Nadel JA (2000) Role of neutrophil elastase in hypersecretion during COPD exacerbations, and proposed therapies. Chest 117:386S–389S
104. Liao SX, Ding T, Rao XM, Sun DS, Sun PP, Wang YJ, Fu DD, Liu XL, Ou-Yang Y (2015) Cigarette smoke affects dendritic cell maturation in the small airways of patients with chronic obstructive pulmonary disease. Mol Med Rep 11(1):219–225
105. Soler P, Moreau A, Basset F et al (1989) Cigarette smoking-induced changes in the number and differentiated state of pulmonary dendritic cells/Langerhans cells. Am Rev Respir Dis 139:1112–1117

106. Demedts IK, Bracke KR, Van Pottelberge G et al (2007) Accumulation of dendritic cells and increased CCL20 levels in the airways of patients with chronic obstructive pulmonary disease. Am J Respir Crit Care Med 175:998–1005
107. Zhuo S, Li N, Zheng Y, Peng X, Xu A, Ge Y (2015) Expression of the lymphocyte chemokine XCL1 in lung tissue of COPD mice, and its relationship to CD4+/CD8+ ratio and IL-2. Cell Biochem Biophys 73:505–511
108. Forsslund H, Mikko M, Karimi R, Grunewald J, Wheelock ÅM, Wahlström J et al (2014) Distribution of T-cell subsets in BAL fluid of patients with mild to moderate COPD depends on current smoking status and not airway obstruction. Chest 145:711–722
109. Roos-Engstrand E, Ekstrand-Hammarstrom B, Pourazar J et al (2009) Influence of smoking cessation on airway T lymphocyte subsets in COPD. COPD 6:112–120
110. Hsu CL, Chhiba KD, Krier-Burris R, Hosakoppal S, Berdnikovs S, Miller ML, Bryce PJ (2020) Allergic inflammation is initiated by IL-33-dependent crosstalk between mast cells and basophils. PLoS One 15(1):e0226701
111. Crivellato E, Travan L, Ribatti D (2015) The phylogenetic profile of mast cells. Methods Mol Biol 1220:11–27
112. Olivera A, Beaven MA, Metcalfe DD (2018) Mast cells signal their importance in health and disease. J Allergy Clin Immunol 142(2):381–393
113. DeBruin EJ, Gold M, Lo BC, Snyder K, Cait A, Lasic N, Lopez M, McNagny KM, Hughes MR (2015) Mast cells in human health and disease. Methods Mol Biol 1220:93–119
114. Pesci A, Rossi A, Bertorelli G, Aufiero A, Zanon P, Olivieri D (1994) Mast cells in the airway lumen and bronchial mucosa of patients with chronic bronchitis. Am J Respir Crit Care Med 149(5):1311–1316
115. Lee B, Kim Y, Kim YM, Jung J, Kim T, Lee SY, Shin YI, Ryu JH (2019) Anti-oxidant and anti-inflammatory effects of aquatic exercise in allergic airway inflammation in mice. Front Physiol 10:1227
116. Mowery PD, Babb S, Hobart R, Tworek C, MacNeil A (2012) The impact of state preemption of local smoking restrictions on public health protections and changes in social norms. J Environ Public Health 2012:632629
117. Stead LF, Buitrago D, Preciado N, Sanchez G, Hartmann-Boyce J, Lancaster T (2013) Physician advice for smoking cessation. Cochrane Database Syst Rev 5:CD000165
118. Jackson SE, McGowan JA, Ubhi HK, Proudfoot H, Shahab L, Brown J, West R (2019) Modelling continuous abstinence rates over time from clinical trials of pharmacological interventions for smoking cessation. Addiction 114(5):787–797
119. Filippidis FT, Laverty AA, Mons U, Jimenez-Ruiz C, Vardavas CI (2019) Changes in smoking cessation assistance in the European Union between 2012 and 2017: pharmacotherapy versus counselling versus e-cigarettes. Tob Control 28(1):95–100
120. Lindson-Hawley N, Hartmann-Boyce J, Fanshawe TR, Begh RB, Farley A, Lancaster T (2016) Interventions to reduce harm from continued tobacco use. Cochrane Database Syst Rev 10:CD005231
121. d'Adesky ND, de Rivero Vaccari JP, Bhattacharya P, Schatz M, Perez-Pinzon MA, Bramlett HM, Raval AP (2018) Nicotine alters estrogen receptor-beta-regulated inflammasome activity and exacerbates ischemic brain damage in female rats. Int J Mol Sci 19(5):1330
122. Sifat AE, Vaidya B, Kaisar MA, Cucullo L, Abbruscato TJ (2018) Nicotine and electronic cigarette (E-Cig) exposure decreases brain glucose utilization in ischemic stroke. J Neurochem 147(2):204–221
123. Herath SC, Normansell R, Maisey S, Poole P (2018) Prophylactic antibiotic therapy for chronic obstructive pulmonary disease (COPD). Cochrane Database Syst Rev 10:CD009764
124. Halpin DMG, Miravitlles M, Metzdorf N, Celli B (2017) Impact and prevention of severe exacerbations of COPD: a review of the evidence. Int J Chron Obstruct Pulmon Dis 12:2891–2908
125. Rogers DF (2007) Mucoactive agents for airway mucus hypersecretory diseases. Respir Care 52(9):1176–1193

126. Poole PJ, Black PN (2012) Mucolytic agents for chronic bronchitis or chronic obstructive pulmonary disease (Cochrane review). Cochrane Database Syst Rev 8:CD001287
127. Rogers DF (2002) Mucoactive drugs for asthma and COPD: any place in therapy? Expert Opin Investig Drugs 11:15–35
128. Rabe KF, Hurd S, Anzueto A, Barnes PJ, Buist SA, Calverley P, Fukuchi Y, Jenkins C, Rodriguez-Roisin R, van Weel C, Zielinski J (2007) Global strategy for the diagnosis, management, and prevention of chronic obstructive pulmonary disease: GOLD executive summary. Am J Respir Crit Care Med 176(6):532–555
129. Hillas G, Perlikos F, Tsiligianni I, Tzanakis N (2015) Managing comorbidities in COPD. Int J Chron Obstruct Pulmon Dis 7(10):95–109
130. Barnes PJ (2013) Theophylline. Am J Respir Crit Care Med 188:901–906
131. Toledo-Pons N, Cosío BG (2017) Is there room for theophylline in COPD? Arch Bronconeumol 53(10):539–540
132. Cosío BG, Shafiek H, Iglesias A, Yanez A, Córdova R, Palou A et al (2016) Oral low-dose theophylline on top of inhaled fluticasone-salmeterol does not reduce exacerbations in patients with severe COPD: a pilot clinical trial. Chest 150:123–130
133. Matera MG, Page CP, Calzetta L, Rogliani P, Cazzola M (2020) Pharmacology and therapeutics of bronchodilators revisited. Pharmacol Rev 72(1):218–252
134. Higgins BG, Powell RM, Cooper S, Tattersfield AE (1991) Effect of salbutamol and ipratropium bromide on airway calibre and bronchial reactivity in asthma and chronic bronchitis. Eur Respir J 4(4):415–420
135. Vathenen AS, Britton JR, Ebden P, Cookson JB, Wharrad HJ, Tattersfield AE (1988) High-dose inhaled albuterol in severe chronic airflow limitation. Am Rev Respir Dis 138 (4):850–855
136. Sestini P, Renzoni E, Robinson S, Poole P, Ram FS (2002) Short-acting beta 2 agonists for stable chronic obstructive pulmonary disease. Cochrane Database Syst Rev 4:CD001495
137. Cazzola M, Rogliani P, Ruggeri P et al (2013) Chronic treatment with indacaterol and airway response to salbutamol in stable COPD. Respir Med 107(6):848–853
138. Kew KM, Mavergames C, Walters JA (2013) Long-acting beta2-agonists for chronic obstructive pulmonary disease. Cochrane Database Syst Rev 10:CD010177
139. Ferguson GT (2000) Update on pharmacologic therapy for chronic obstructive pulmonary disease. Clin Chest Med 21:723–738
140. Melani AS (2015) Long-acting muscarinic antagonists. Exp Rev Clin Pharmacol 8 (4):479–501
141. Karner C, Chong J, Poole P (2014) Tiotropium versus placebo for chronic obstructive pulmonary disease. Cochrane Database Syst Rev 7:CD009285
142. Disse B, Speck GA, Rominger KL, Witek TJ Jr, Hammer R (1999) Tiotropium (Spiriva): mechanistical considerations and clinical profile in obstructive lung disease. Life Sci 64 (6-7):457–464
143. Kesten S, Jara M, Wentworth C, Lanes S (2006) Pooled clinical trial analysis of tiotropium safety. Chest 130(6):1695–1703
144. Anthonisen NR, Connett JE, Enright PL, Manfreda J, Lung Health Study Research G (2002) Hospitalizations and mortality in the Lung Health Study. Am J Respir Crit Care Med 166 (3):333–339
145. Rao F, Chen Z, Zhou D, Kang Y, Guo L, Xue YJ (2018) DFT investigation on the metabolic mechanisms of theophylline by cytochrome P450 monooxygenase. Mol Graph Model 84:109–117
146. Matera MG, Page C, Cazzola M (2017) Doxofylline is not just another theophylline! Int J Chron Obstruct Pulmon Dis 5(12):3487–3493
147. Abdulai RM, Jensen TJ, Patel NR, Polkey MI, Jansson P, Celli BR, Rennard SI (2018) Deterioration of limb muscle function during acute exacerbation of chronic obstructive pulmonary disease. Am J Respir Crit Care Med 197(4):433–449

148. Rabe KF, Calverley PMA, Martinez FJ, Fabbri LM (2017) Effect of roflumilast in patients with severe COPD and a history of hospitalisation. Eur Respir J 50(1):1700158
149. Yang IA, Clarke MS, Sim EH, Fong KM (2012) Inhaled corticosteroids for stable chronic obstructive pulmonary disease. Cochrane Database Syst Rev 7:CD002991
150. Mahler DA, Kerwin E, Ayers T et al (2015) FLIGHT1 and FLIGHT2: efficacy and safety of QVA149 (indacaterol/glycopyrrolate) versus its monocomponents and placebo in patients with chronic obstructive pulmonary disease. Am J Respir Crit Care Med 192(9):1068–1079
151. Cazzola M, Molimard M (2010) The scientific rationale for combining long-acting beta2-agonists and muscarinic antagonists in COPD. Pulm Pharmacol Ther 23(4):257–267
152. Gross N, Tashkin D, Miller R, Oren J, Coleman W, Linberg S (1998) Inhalation by nebulization of albuterolipratropium combination (Dey combination) is superior to either agent alone in the treatment of chronic obstructive pulmonary disease. Dey Combination Solution Study Group. Respiration 65(5):354–362
153. Tashkin DP, Pearle J, Iezzoni D, Varghese ST (2009) Formoterol and tiotropium compared with tiotropium alone for treatment of COPD. COPD 6(1):17–25
154. Nannini LJ, Lasserson TJ, Poole P (2012) Combined corticosteroid and long-acting beta(2)-agonist in one inhaler versus long-acting beta(2)-agonists for chronic obstructive pulmonary disease. Cochrane Database Syst Rev 9:CD006829
155. Nannini LJ, Poole P, Milan SJ, Kesterton A (2013) Combined corticosteroid and long-acting beta(2)-agonist in one inhaler versus inhaled corticosteroids alone for chronic obstructive pulmonary disease. Cochrane Database Syst Rev 8:CD006826
156. Brusselle G, Price D, Gruffydd-Jones K et al (2015) The inevitable drift to triple therapy in COPD: an analysis of prescribing pathways in the UK. Int J Chron Obstruct Pulmon Dis 10:2207–2217
157. Jung KS, Park HY, Park SY et al (2012) Comparison of tiotropium plus fluticasone propionate/salmeterol with tiotropium in COPD: a randomized controlled study. Respir Med 106 (3):382–389
158. Hanania NA, Crater GD, Morris AN, Emmett AH, O'Dell DM, Niewoehner DE (2012) Benefits of adding fluticasone propionate/salmeterol to tiotropium in moderate to severe COPD. Respir Med 106(1):91–101
159. Stoller JK, Aboussouan LS (2012) A review of alpha1-antitrypsin deficiency. Am J Respir Crit Care Med 185(3):246–259
160. Sandhaus R, Turino G, Brantly M et al (2016) The diagnosis and management of alpha-1 antitrypsin deficiency in the adult. Chronic Obstr Pulm Dis 3(3):668–682
161. Wu DD, Song J, Bartel S, Krauss-Etschmann S, Rots MG, Hylkema MN (2018) The potential for targeted rewriting of epigenetic marks in COPD as a new therapeutic approach. Pharmacol Ther 182:1–14
162. Wattiez R, Falmagne P (2005) Proteomics of bronchoalveolar lavage fluid. J Chromatogr B Analyt Technol Biomed Life Sci 815(1-2):169–178
163. Maltesen RG, Buggeskov KB, Andersen CB, Plovsing R, Wimmer R, Ravn HB, Rasmussen BS (2018) Lung protection strategies during cardiopulmonary bypass affect the composition of bronchoalveolar fluid and lung tissue in cardiac surgery patients. Metabolites 8(4):E54
164. Wu J, Kobayashi M, Sousa EA, Liu W, Cai J, Goldman SJ, Dorner AJ, Projan SJ, Kavuru MS, Qiu Y, Thomassen MJ (2005) Differential proteomic analysis of bronchoalveolar lavage fluid in asthmatics following segmental antigen challenge. Mol Cell Proteomics 4(9):1251–1264
165. Terracciano R, Preiano M, Palladino GP, Carpagnano GE et al (2011) Peptidome profiling of induced sputum by mesoporous silica beads and MALDI-TOF MS for non-invasive biomarker discovery of chronic inflammatory lung diseases. Proteomics 11:3402–3414
166. Savino R, Terracciano R (2012) Mesopore-assisted profiling strategies in clinical proteomics for drug/target discovery. Drug Discov Today 17:143–152
167. Auffray C, Adcock IM, Chung KF, Djukanovic R et al (2010) An integrative systems biology approach to understanding pulmonary diseases. Chest 137:1410–1416
168. Nicholas BL, O'Connor CD, Djukanovic R (2009) From proteomics to prescription-the search for COPD biomarkers. COPD 6:298–303

The manufacturer's authorised representative in the EU is Springer Nature Customer Service Centre GmbH, Europaplatz 3, 69115 Heidelberg, Germany. If you have any concerns regarding our products, please contact ProductSafety@springernature.com

Printed and bound by CPI Group (UK) Ltd, Croydon, CR0 4YY

30/07/2026

02181626-0005